Is Evidence-based Psychiatry Ethical?

International Perspectives in Philosophy and Psychiatry

Series editors: Bill (K.W.M.) Fulford, Lisa Bortolotti, Matthew Broome, Katherine Morris, John Z. Sadler, and Giovanni Stanghellini

Volumes in the series:

Portrait of the Psychiatrist as a Young Man: The Early Writing and Work of R.D. Laing, 1927–1960
Beveridge

Mind, Meaning, and Mental Disorder 2e
Bolton and Hill

What is Mental Disorder?
Bolton

Delusions and Other Irrational Beliefs
Bortolotti

Postpsychiatry
Bracken and Thomas

Philosophy, Psychoanalysis, and the A-Rational Mind
Brakel

Unconscious Knowing and Other Essays in Psycho-Philosophical Analysis
Brakel

Psychiatry as Cognitive Neuroscience
Broome and Bortolotti (eds.)

Free Will and Responsibility: A Guide for Practitioners
Callender

Reconceiving Schizophrenia
Chung, Fulford, and Graham (eds.)

Darwin and Psychiatry
De Block and Adriaens (eds.)

Oxford Handbook of Philosophy and Psychiatry
Fulford, Davies, Gipps, Graham, Sadler, Stanghellini, and Thornton

Nature and Narrative: An Introduction to the New Philosophy of Psychiatry
Fulford, Morris, Sadler, and Stanghellini (eds.)

Oxford Textbook of Philosophy and Psychiatry
Fulford, Thornton, and Graham

The Mind and its Discontents
Gillett

Thinking Through Dementia
Hughes

Dementia: Mind, Meaning, and the Person
Hughes, Louw, and Sabat (eds.)

Talking Cures and Placebo Effects
Jopling

Philosophical Issues in Psychiatry II: Nosology
Kendler and Parnas (eds.)

Discursive Perspectives in Therapeutic Practice
Lock and Strong (eds.)

Schizophrenia and the Fate of the Self
Lysaker and Lysaker

Responsibility and Psychopathy
Malatesti and McMillan

Body-Subjects and Disordered Minds
Matthews

Rationality and Compulsion: Applying Action Theory to Psychiatry
Nordenfelt

Philosophical Perspectives on Technology and Psychiatry
Phillips (ed.)

The Metaphor of Mental Illness
Pickering

Mapping the Edges and the In-between
Potter

Trauma, Truth, and Reconciliation: Healing Damaged Relationships
Potter (ed.)

The Philosophy of Psychiatry: A Companion
Radden

The Virtuous Psychiatrist
Radden and Sadler

Addiction and Weakness of Will
Radoilska

Autonomy and Mental Disorder
Radoilska (ed.)

Feelings of Being
Ratcliffe

Recovery of People with Mental Illness: Philosophical and Related Perspectives
Rudnick (ed.)

Values and Psychiatric Diagnosis
Sadler

Disembodied Spirits and Deanimated Bodies: The Psychopathology of Common Sense
Stanghellini

One Century of Karl Jaspers' Psychopathology
Stanghellini and Fuchs (eds.)

Emotions and Personhood
Stanghellini and Rosfort

Essential Philosophy of Psychiatry
Thornton

Empirical Ethics in Psychiatry
Widdershoven, McMillan, Hope, and Van der Scheer (eds.)

The Sublime Object of Psychiatry: Schizophrenia in Clinical and Cultural Theory
Woods

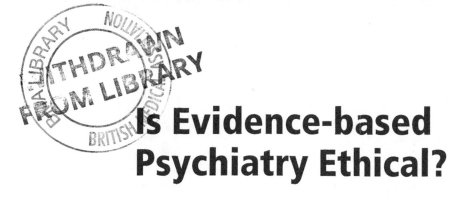

Is Evidence-based Psychiatry Ethical?

Mona Gupta

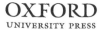
OXFORD
UNIVERSITY PRESS

OXFORD
UNIVERSITY PRESS

Great Clarendon Street, Oxford, OX2 6DP,
United Kingdom

Oxford University Press is a department of the University of Oxford.
It furthers the University's objective of excellence in research, scholarship,
and education by publishing worldwide. Oxford is a registered trade mark of
Oxford University Press in the UK and in certain other countries

First Edition published in 2014

Impression: 1

Published in the United States of America by Oxford University Press
198 Madison Avenue, New York, NY 10016, United States of America

British Library Cataloguing in Publication Data
Data available

Library of Congress Control Number: 2014933290

ISBN 978–0–19–964111–6

Printed in Great Britain by
Clays Ltd., St Ives plc

To my patients

Acknowledgements

Writing this book was both an engaging and a demanding experience, in all of the ways that make academic life rich and rewarding. It was, admittedly, less glamorous than I had imagined, with long hours spent in my windowless basement, dressed in track pants, and surrounded by unpacked boxes from a house move that had occurred two years previously. But these temporary inconveniences were minor compared to the contributions of so many people who have helped me along the way.

The book began its life as my doctoral dissertation, completed at the University of Toronto. I owe a debt of gratitude to my thesis committee for their unfailing support and guidance: Ross Upshur (my supervisor), Bill Harvey, Lynne Lohfeld, and Lawrie Reznek. Anthony Levitt was my department chief during these years. He believed in me and his support enabled me to fulfil my dream of having a career in academic medicine.

The research that formed the basis of this book could not have been completed without the research participants, who gave their time generously and trusted me with their insights. The Canadian Institutes of Health Research provided invaluable financial support. Bill Fulford, editor of the IPPP series, has been a mentor from the start. Martin Baum and Charlotte Green at Oxford University Press (UK) offered the correct proportions of persistence and patience. Robyn Bluhm, Suzanne Leclair, Nancy Potter, John Sadler, and Peter Zachar unhesitatingly reviewed various chapters and provided detailed and constructive feedback.

I am very grateful for the extensive moral and material support I have received during my career. I had just started writing the book when I moved from Toronto to Montréal to the Centre Hospitalier de l'Université de Montréal (CHUM). My colleagues there welcomed me warmly and maintained a regular supply of optimism and chocolate, encouraging me at every turn. The CHUM's Department of Psychiatry and Centre de Recherche, as well as the Department of Psychiatry of the University of Montréal, have supported me as a clinician-investigator, both valuing and promoting the humanities in psychiatry.

My parents, Mohini and Jagdish Gupta, supported my education and always encouraged my career. My mother, a political scientist, understood the significance of 'the book'. My late father, an indefatigable surgeon, underlined the importance of being first and foremost a clinician. My brother Nalin, himself an academic surgeon, has been a powerful, positive example of how to combine clinical practice and research.

My husband and children are the bedrock of my life. They made it possible to persevere with the project and to forge on in my working life. Naomi, Neil and Gopika, you fill every corner of my life with joy. David, there is no way to enumerate the thousands of ways you have helped and supported me in our life together, although the double espressos, apple martinis, and frequent primers on the history of psychiatry deserve special mention. Quite simply, thank you for everything. I could never have done this without you.

Contents

1 What does evidence have to do with ethics? *1*

2 What is evidence-based medicine? *13*

3 Values and evidence-based medicine: the debate *45*

4 Psychiatry and evidence-based psychiatry *69*

5 The critique of evidence-based psychiatry *91*

6 The ethics of evidence-based medicine *117*

7 Experts talk about ethics, evidence-based medicine, and psychiatry *149*

8 Is evidence-based psychiatric practice ethical? *167*

9 Conclusions *181*

Appendix 1 *187*
Index *197*

Chapter 1

What does evidence have to do with ethics?

'Pinel did not cut the chains of the mentally ill because he had just read a well-controlled randomized trial on the effect of chains.'

Participant 2-10[1]

1.1 Why a Book about Evidence-Based Medicine and Ethics?

Over the last hundred years, medical research has led to a vast expansion in our knowledge about the human body and its diseases. At the same time, there have been significant developments in the treatments for many health conditions. As a result, we believe firmly that medical research is the route to further knowledge, and further knowledge leads to better health. In recent years, this direct connection between research, knowledge, and improved health has been famously articulated in the concept of evidence-based medicine (EBM). Developed in the early 1990s at McMaster University, EBM is defined as '... the conscientious, explicit, and judicious use of current best evidence in making decisions about the care of individual patients' (Guyatt et al. 2008: 783).

EBM captures a very simple and compelling principle—that clinical decision-making should be based, as much as possible, on the most up-to-date research findings. In order to determine which research data offer the best evidence concerning health care interventions, EBM relies on a ranking of research methods from those most likely to those least likely to support truthful conclusions about these interventions. This hierarchy determines which studies yield the best evidence, based on whether they have employed the highest-ranked methods.

But why should we think that EBM, a movement devoted to increasing the knowledge behind clinical decision-making, has something to do with ethics?

---

[1] For a description of the anonymization of participants, see Section 1.3.

Even though EBM's primary claim is an empirical one—that adhering to EBM will lead to improvements in health outcomes—there is no evidence of the kind preferred by EBM that it can achieve this goal, a point which its proponents concede (Haynes 2002; Straus and McAlister 2000). In the absence of evidence that EBM is the best way to practise, EBM is forced to justify itself in another manner, which it does through an implicit, normative claim: that we should practise EBM. EBM assumes that adhering to its principles is the best way to obtain knowledge about which medical interventions are effective and, therefore, is the best path to improving health. To practise anything but EBM would knowingly lead patients to less effective interventions and worse health. Such a state of affairs could not count as good practice. Thus, EBM's implicit justification is also an ethical one: we should practise EBM because it is the best (most accurate) way to help patients achieve improved health.

Increasingly, good practice (both technically and ethically speaking) is becoming synonymous with evidence-based practice[2]. Yet, there are other ethically relevant considerations in clinical decision-making apart from what is likely to lead to the kinds of health outcomes typically evaluated by clinical research studies. This book looks at where such considerations fit, if at all, in the practice of EBM.

1.2 Why a Book about EBM, Ethics, and Psychiatry?

Many of EBM's leading authors trained in internal medicine and originally envisioned several of its principles applied to problems in their field. Some of the leading EBM online resources, such as *UpToDate*[3] and *Clinical Evidence*,[4] started out with many more entries related to topics in internal medicine than, for example, to psychiatry. But EBM's popularity has spread beyond internal medicine to other clinical disciplines, including psychiatry (Geddes and Harrison 1997; Paris 2000).

In fact, evidence-based psychiatry—the straightforward application of the principles of EBM to the practice of psychiatry (Gupta 2007)—has received enthusiastic endorsement from professional societies representing psychiatrists in many countries. Why might this be so? Both popular and scholarly

---

[2] At times I use the term 'evidence-based practice', by which I mean simply using the EBM method in clinical practice.

[3] *UpToDate*® is an online resource that offers a searchable encyclopaedia of reviews of clinical topics. It is provided by Wolters Kluwer Health and is available by paid subscription.

[4] *Clinical Evidence* is a database of overviews assessing the benefits and harms of treatments. It is provided by BMJ Publishing Group Limited and is available by paid subscription.

depictions of the harms done to patients in the name of psychiatric treatment continue to have a widespread negative influence on public opinion (Kesey 1968; Szasz 1974). And because the pathophysiological basis of mental disorders remains unknown, this further damages psychiatry's claim to being a legitimate medical discipline. If we don't know why people develop mental disorders, then on what basis can psychiatrists distinguish between illness and normalcy? Are these distinctions based on true knowledge or merely the beliefs and values of psychiatrists? By contrast, the ethical value of other medical specialties is rarely in doubt—people do not question society's need to devote vast resources to oncology; lobby groups do not spring up opposing gastroenterology; there has never been an antidermatology movement (as there is an antipsychiatry movement). It is into the context of this ethical debate about psychiatry that EBM enters. Advocates of an evidence-based approach to psychiatry hope that, if practice is driven by hard scientific data rather than the traditions and inferences characteristic of past eras, there will be greater potential to improve patients' health (Szatmari 2003; Goldner et al. 2001). This, in turn, will solidify psychiatry as a scientifically legitimate and ethical medical practice in the minds of the patients, policy-makers, and psychiatrists themselves.

What is the relationship between ethical practice and evidence-based practice in medicine and in psychiatry, exactly? The literature on the relationship between ethics and EBM tends to focus on the ethical consequences of using or not using best evidence in practice. Goldenberg argues that interrogating the relationship between ethics and EBM should reach beyond the consequences of using EBM in practice and investigate the ways that ethical values are relevant to the generation of evidence (knowledge production) (2007: 62–3). Such an expansion would encourage examination of the contextual values that are part of the social context in which EBM operates. Several scholars have pointed out that ethical values, either implicit or explicit, operate at all phases of research—not only the generation but also the dissemination and interpretation of data (Downie et al. 2000; Eysenck 1994; Gilbody and Song 2000). These values include judgements about which research questions and health outcomes should be studied and/or funded for study; how to study and represent certain outcomes (e.g. how one should represent a change in depression); which conclusions ought to be presented, published, and emphasized; and how data ought to be situated within the larger body of clinical knowledge (e.g. when there are enough data to change practice or insurance coverage).

Because any approach to clinical knowledge orientates us towards what we ought to know about health, and because health is tied to human flourishing, the very notion of what counts as evidence is not only a matter of fact but also one of ethics. Therefore, in addition to contextual or external values, an exploration of the ethics of EBM must also consider internal values. Such considerations would include, for example, how choices about research methods influence what we can know and, therefore, value about health; and how we determine what counts as evidence about health. In other words, there are ethical implications of EBM, but it may also be constituted by certain ethical values (Borgerson 2008: 40–1).

Evidence-based psychiatry is equally implicated in this general analysis of the relationship between ethical practice and evidence-based practice. However, there are specific reasons to be concerned about the ethics of evidence-based psychiatry. Emerging as it did with internal medicine in mind (and the large-scale clinical trials of pharmaceutical agents), EBM makes certain assumptions about the nature of disease that may not be applicable to psychiatric disorders, or their treatments. To the extent that psychiatric disorders do not conform to these assumptions, the application of EBM to psychiatry is more likely to be fraught with epistemological and ethical problems than its application to other branches of medicine.

Does making psychiatry evidence-based strengthen its scientific, and therefore its ethical credibility? Whether the application of EBM to psychiatry really does offer improved scientific substantiation to psychiatric knowledge remains controversial. Given the longstanding debates about the use and abuse of power in psychiatry (Foucault 1973; Szasz 1974), using dubious knowledge claims under the guise of doing what's best for patients may be ethically suspect.

Is evidence-based psychiatric practice, ethical? This book aims to answer this question. Therefore, it does not focus on the ways that EBM dovetails with other clinically related spheres such as health policy or medical education. These are important areas in their own right, requiring their own analyses. In this book I wish to focus attention on the very context for which EBM was originally conceived: the individual doctor–patient encounter. Some of the ethical concerns discussed are common to all health disciplines where EBM has been utilized. Others are particular to psychiatry, given the unique subject matter of that field and the persistent debates about its ethical legitimacy as a specialty of medicine.

1.3 The Argument Ahead

In exploring and defining the relationship between ethics and evidence-based psychiatry, the book draws upon two primary sources. The first is the two authoritative texts that lay out the principles and methods of EBM—namely, Guyatt et al.'s *Users' guides to the medical literature: a manual for evidence-based clinical practice* (2nd edition, 2008, hereafter *Users' guides*) and Straus et al.'s *Evidence-based medicine: how to practice and teach it* (4th edition, 2011, hereafter *Evidence-based medicine*). The second set of sources is made up of interviews that I conducted with three groups of respondents: group 1 consisted of nine people who were, and remain, involved in the development of EBM (referred to as 'EBM developers'); group 2 consisted of 11 practitioners working in mental health, who are involved in the implementation and scholarly debate about the use of EBM in mental health practice (referred to as 'mental health experts'); and group 3 included 13 scholars who have investigated philosophical or ethical aspects of EBM (referred to as 'philosophers/bioethicists' or simply 'philosophers'). All group one and two participants were or have been engaged in clinical practice, while only three group three participants had ever worked as clinicians.[5] The EBM texts offer a (sometimes incomplete) picture of EBM. However, because EBM is an approach that continues to evolve, it is necessary to supplement the texts with the ideas expressed by its originators and those engaged in its ongoing development or critique. Other voices in the debate about the ethics of EBM are included in my review of the existing literature in this area.

1.3.1 Contentious Issues

The main question of the book invites the consideration of several basic concepts such as evidence, medicine, health, and mental disorder. Indeed, these concepts relate to even more basic philosophical debates concerning the nature of minds, the justification of knowledge, and the relationship between ethics and epistemology. These important debates form the necessary background, but a philosophical examination of each is beyond the scope of this book. What I have tried to do is illustrate some of the contentious issues that arise in the philosophical debates about these concepts, particularly as they relate to the field of psychiatry and EBM. Given that these component concepts have themselves generated vast philosophical analyses, it will be unsurprising that EBM proves to be a contested idea, both in the literature and among those most expert in its meaning and use. Nevertheless, this lack of clarity surrounding

---

[5] In this book I quote many participants directly, using a numerical code to denote each participant. The first number refers to a participant's disciplinary group (1, 2 or 3). The second number distinguishes each participant from the others within the group. Thus, P1-8 is the eighth participant from group 1. I had to include my question in some quotations in order to contextualize the participant's answer. In these cases, I denote my speech with I (for interviewer) and then quote myself directly. Occasionally I insert text in square brackets; this is usually to clarify an indefinite pronoun.

the concept of EBM exposes some of what is assumed about these more basic concepts when EBM is applied to psychiatric practice.

1.3.2 Defining Terms

The objective of Chapter 2 is to define terms and examine the basic concepts of EBM as depicted in EBM's two authoritative texts: *Users' guides* and *Evidence-based medicine*. The most important of these terms are 'evidence-based medicine' and 'evidence'. I also examine the five steps that comprise the practice of EBM, which its authors describe as a framework for clinical decision-making.

In defining these terms and describing the five steps, the book remains as close to the programmatic descriptions as possible by drawing almost exclusively upon the original texts as source material. I then make use of my interviews with EBM experts to try to further delineate the concept of EBM—what it implies and what it is trying to convey—in order to fill in details missing in the texts. I provide excerpts from the interviews interspersed with my own interpretations of these segments. I also highlight areas of convergence, divergence, and ambiguity between the respondents and the texts, and between respondents themselves. Near the end of the chapter I return to steps 3 and 4, critical appraisal and integration, in an attempt to clarify how EBM works in practice.

1.3.3 Debating EBM

Chapter 3 reviews the debate that has emerged in the scholarly literature, particularly as it concerns EBM's basic concepts and its practice. This review draws attention to several contentious areas relating to EBM's five steps, including the social context of medical research; what kinds of data do, and should, count as evidence; the process by which data become evidence (and evidence for what exactly?); and how evidence becomes meaningfully integrated with clinicians' expertise and patients' values, as EBM instructs that it should. The issues highlighted in this debate, along with the conceptual clarifications of Chapter 2, show how some of the most urgent concerns in the debate about EBM involve the role of ethical values in both its theory and practice.

1.3.4 Applying EBM to Psychiatry

In Chapter 4 I examine concepts that are relevant to applying EBM to psychiatry, including psychiatry, mental disorder, and treatment. The first section of Chapter 4 discusses the evolution of the modern discipline of psychiatry and the assumptions about the nature of mind, disease and treatment that are embedded within its practice. This section argues that current psychiatric practice is framed by the unresolved philosophical debate about the nature of mind.

Psychiatry, as a practical discipline, does not attempt to resolve this debate, even though various theoretical commitments are implied through its diagnostic and treatment practices.

The second section of Chapter 4 defines evidence-based psychiatry. It then returns to the interviewees, who offer their own conceptions of evidence-based psychiatry, compared to what is currently portrayed in mainstream literature. In the third section the interviewees explore the application of EBM to psychiatric diagnosis and treatment. This section argues that adopting EBM leads psychiatry to take on EBM's assumptions about disease and treatment, thereby cementing a commitment to a particular theory of mind and mental experience.

1.3.5 Questioning EBM's Assumptions

In Chapter 5 I examine the ways in which the assumptions about disease and treatment that underlie EBM do and do not apply to mental disorders. Drawing on the academic literature on this point, the first section of this chapter examines the application of EBM to psychiatry, including practical considerations such as the limitations of the way that randomized controlled trials (RCTs) in psychiatry are currently conducted, as well as the difficulties in studying non-pharmacological treatments.

The second and third sections of the chapter discuss several problems that emerge in the clinical research literature in psychiatry, including the placebo effect, the presence of the so-called non-specific therapeutic factors, and the meaning of quantifying mental health outcomes. The chapter concludes by arguing that adopting EBM, which seems to put psychiatry on firmer scientific and ethical ground, leads the field to commit itself to a particular version of mental disorder and treatment, one that is narrower than what is allowed by its current theoretical pluralism.

1.3.6 Ethical Values Embedded in EBM

The first section of Chapter 6 explores the ethical values embedded in EBM's five steps. It goes on to argue that EBM substantiates itself ethically by claiming that it is the best way to achieve health. It then discusses the ethical theory reflected by this stance. This analysis enables me to offer a picture of the ethics of 'literal' EBM—that is, the version of EBM described in its key texts.

In the second section of Chapter 6 I discuss how the ethics of EBM applies to psychiatry. Looking at some clinical examples of diagnosis and treatment, I argue that the ethical values of EBM affect psychiatric practice in distinct ways, given the controversial history of its science and the contested nature of psychiatric disorders themselves.

1.3.7 Important Themes about Ethics and EBM

Chapter 7 returns to the interviewees, discussing four important themes or issues emerging from their views about the relationship of ethics to EBM. The first is that EBM is an exemplar of larger ethical trends in society. The second is whether EBM is value-free or value-laden. The third is how one determines which of EBM's two distinct goals—improved health outcomes versus satisfying patients' preferences—takes priority? The fourth is whether it is or is not ethical that EBM be used as a tool for resource allocation.

Using these themes and example offered by the interviewees, I discuss the relationship between ethical practice and evidence-based practice. Evidence-based practice may or may not be ethical; non-evidence-based practice may or may not be ethical. Whether it is or not depends on certain features of the situation, such as local attitudes to health care, practitioners' values, and patients' psychological needs in the trajectory of their illness. This discussion allows me to use the interviewees' reflections to offer a picture of the enriched ethics of EBM compared to the ethics of literal EBM implied by its foundational texts.

1.3.8 A Last Look at the Ethics of Evidence-based Psychiatry

Chapter 8 addresses the main question of the book: is evidence-based psychiatric practice, ethical? While psychiatrists hoped that EBM could help to solidity its scientific and ethical credentials, in Chapter 5 we saw that this may not be possible. If EBM cannot supply psychiatry with the ethical substantiation it seeks, what will do the job? This chapter contrasts EBM's ethics with those underlying several other approaches to the clinical encounter, including the biopsychosocial model, postpsychiatry, and values-based practice.

I conclude by taking a last look at the ethics of EBM. Does it have something distinct to offer psychiatry? I argue that quite apart from its utilitarian impulses, EBM contains an implicit call to virtue. That is, it asks clinicians to cultivate the intellectual and moral virtues involved in responsible scientific knowing. This may be EBM's most important and innovative contribution to ethical, clinical practice.

1.3.9 Future Directions

Where does a clearer understanding of the ethics of evidence-based psychiatry leave the field, and in what directions does psychiatry need to evolve scientifically and ethically? I offer three conclusions following the arguments made in this book. The first is that EBM could be improved if it were to contract: aim to do a smaller task that would be at once more modest but also more defensible, epistemologically and ethically. The second conclusion is that psychiatry needs to reject the constraining discourse of EBM and define the questions and methods that are appropriate to the subject material of its discipline—whether these are or are not part of the subject matter of the rest of medicine. The third conclusion is that by identifying how and where ethical values play a role in psychiatric practice, bioethical analysis offers psychiatry a helpful companion. The question is not whether ethical values are at play in psychiatry, but whose values and why?

Does psychiatry need to stake out its own ground, scientifically and ethically, compared with other medical specialties, in order to best respond to the particular characteristics of mental disorders and the needs of those who suffer from them? If so, what would that look like? This type of discussion goes beyond the debate about EBM towards the development of psychiatry's own vision of ethical, clinical practice.

1.3.10 Overall Methodological Approach

The appendix offers a detailed description of the overall methodological approach for the interviews and the techniques used, as well as a discussion of the interpretative framework that was brought to bear upon the interviews. I review the ethical considerations for the interviewees, including the process of obtaining informed consent, and protection of confidentiality and anonymity.

1.4 Interpretive Considerations

My goal in writing this book is to examine evidence-based psychiatry using the perspective and methods of bioethics, in the hope that this will deepen the understanding of the issues psychiatrists face in trying to practise EBM. I hope that the content will resonate with clinicians as well as those scholars within bioethics and philosophy who work on subjects related to clinical practice.

I have tried to offer a faithful and honest rendering of the foundational texts that describe EBM. When it comes to ethics, some of the arguments are implied. At times I discuss what is implied in the texts, particularly when it is supported by the interpretations of other authors or EBM authors' other writings. However, much of what we want to know about the ethics of EBM is left unsaid. In this case, I do not try to guess the authors' meaning or read between the lines but simply leave certain ideas in the original wording, pointing out where detail or explanation is lacking.

Meanwhile, the reader should be aware where my personal sympathies, biases, and beliefs as a researcher lie. I came to this project as a critic of EBM myself, sympathetic to arguments expressing concern about the epistemologi-cal underpinnings of EBM.

Because I interviewed most of the EBM developers first, my own beliefs about EBM were challenged at an early stage of the project. Trying to adopt-ing the neutral stance of an interviewer required me to evaluate the 'pro-EBM' arguments more dispassionately and reflect more deeply on their meaning. As I went on to interview mental health practitioners and philosophers/bioethi-cists, I saw how nuanced their critical views were. The terms 'proponent' and 'critic' did not fully capture the sophistication of their arguments and instead created a black and white frame to the debate. Nevertheless, I have retained the use of these terms at various points to reflect the fact that, despite the nuance, there are experts who believe wholeheartedly in EBM and others who wish to see it abandoned, or at least greatly modified.

References

Borgerson, K. (2008), 'Valuing and evaluating evidence in medicine', PhD thesis, University of Toronto.

Downie, R. S. and MacNaughton, J. with Randall, F. (2000), 'Judgment and science', in: *Clinical judgment: evidence in practice* (New York: Oxford University Press), 1–39.

Eysenck, H. (1994), 'Meta-analysis and its problems', *British Medical Journal*, **309**: 789–92.

Foucault, M. (1973), *Madness and civilization*, tr. R. Howard (New York: Random House).

Geddes, J. R. and Harrison, P.J. (1997), 'Closing the gap between research and practice', *British Journal of Psychiatry*, **171**: 220–5.

Gilbody, S. M. and Song, F. (2000), 'Publication bias and the integrity of psychiatry research', *Psychological Medicine*, **30**: 253–8.

Goldenberg, M. (2007), 'Advancing an ethics of evidence: a critical appraisal of evidence based medicine and feminist theories of evidence', PhD thesis, University of Michigan.

Goldner, E. M., Abbass, A., Leverette, J. S., and Haslam, D. R. (2001), 'Evidence-based psychiatric practice: implications for education and continuing professional develop-ment', *Canadian Journal of Psychiatry*, **46**: 424–39.

Gupta, M. (2007), 'Does evidence-based medicine apply to psychiatry?', *Theoretical Medicine and Bioethics*, **28**: 103–20.

Guyatt, G., Rennie, D., Meade, M., and Cook, D. (2008) (eds.), *Users' guides to the medical literature: a manual for evidence-based clinical practice*, 2nd edn. (Chicago: AMA Press).

Haynes, R. B. (2002), 'What kind of evidence is it that evidence-based medicine advocates want health care providers and consumers to pay attention to?', *BMC Health Services Research*, **2** (3): March 6 <http://www.biomedcentral.com/1472-6963/2/3> accessed 28 January 2014.

Kesey, K. (1968, first pub. 1962), *One flew over the cuckoo's nest: a novel* (New York: Viking Press).

Paris, J. (2000), 'Canadian psychiatry across 5 decades: from clinical inference to evidence-based practice', *Canadian Journal of Psychiatry*, **45**: 34–9.

Straus, S. E. and McAlister, F. A. (2000), 'Evidence-based medicine: a commentary on common criticisms', *Canadian Medical Association Journal*, **163**: 837–41.

Straus, S. E., Richardson, W. S., Glasziou, P., and Haynes, R. B. (2011) (eds.), *Evidence-based medicine: how to practice and teach EBM*, 4th edn. (Edinburgh: Elsevier Churchill Livingstone).

Szasz, T. S. (1974), *The myth of mental illness* (New York: Harper and Row).

Szatmari, P. (2003), 'The art of evidence-based child psychiatry', *Evidence-Based Mental Health*, **6**: 1–3.

Chapter 2

What is evidence-based medicine?

2.1 Definition

In only 20 years the concept of evidence-based medicine (EBM) has captured the imagination of the medical world. Coined in 1990 by Gordon Guyatt, then the director of residency training for internal medicine at McMaster University in Hamilton, Ontario, Canada, the phrase first appeared in an information document for prospective applicants to the residency programme (Guyatt et al. 2008: xxi). Guyatt was searching for a phrase to capture the methods of teaching and practising medicine that he, and several colleagues, had been developing at McMaster over the previous decade.

These methods emerged from the work of David Sackett and colleagues in the Department of Clinical Epidemiology and Biostatistics at McMaster. Sackett, a specialist in internal medicine and founding chair of the department, had written a textbook in 1985 about clinical epidemiology and its applications to clinical research. With colleagues from the department, Sackett wanted to share his knowledge of research methods with the average practitioner. He believed that if practitioners were better equipped to understand medical research, they would be more likely to draw upon recent findings in clinical decision-making. In his view, so they should, as this would improve the care they offered. To that end, he and his colleagues published an influential series of guides to reading the medical literature in the *Canadian Medical Association Journal*; these appeared between 1981 and 1984. Brian Haynes (another specialist in internal medicine in the department) and colleagues published a related series in the *Annals of Internal Medicine* in 1986.

A 1992 article in the *Journal of the American Medical Association* (*JAMA*) introduced the concept of EBM to the medical world and defined it as '. . . the conscientious, explicit, and judicious use of current best evidence in making decisions about the care of individual patients' (Evidence-Based Medicine Working Group, 1992). From these origins, the concept has become enormously influential in medical education, clinical practice, and health policy (Grossman and McKenzie 2005: 6; Ghali et al. 1999: 133–4; Noseworthy and Watanabe 1999: 230). For example, teaching medical students and residents the basic principles of critical appraisal (part of the EBM method) is now commonplace, while policy-makers commonly claim that they must ensure the population has access to evidence-based interventions. Although its originators were primarily practitioners of internal medicine, EBM has been taken up throughout the medical specialties and the allied health disciplines. In 2007 the *British Medical Journal* included EBM among a list of 15 of the most important discoveries in medicine since 1840 (Morrison 2007). EBM has even extended its reach to the popular press. In 2001, the *New York Times Magazine* voted EBM one of the best ideas of the year (Hitt 2001).

2.1.1 **Textbooks of EBM**

The concept of EBM is by no means static. It continues to evolve and many of its originators remain actively involved in its development. These authors have, with additional collaborators, produced and revised two authoritative textbooks of EBM. The first, *Evidence-based medicine: how to practice and teach EBM*,[1] was originally authored by Sackett, Richardson, Rosenberg and Haynes in 1997, and is now in its fourth edition. The current edition (2011) was written by four authors—Straus, Glasziou, Richardson, and Haynes. Sackett, lead author on the first two editions, did not contribute thereafter.[2] The second textbook is *Users' guides to the medical literature*,[3] penned by the 50-member Evidence-Based Medicine Working Group. *Users' guides* is an edited collection of a series of articles under the same title that appeared in *JAMA* between 1992 and 2000. It is now in its second edition (2008). All the present authors of *Evidence-based medicine* contributed to *Users' guides*. Given the authorial overlap, there is general consistency between the texts. In fact, *Evidence-based medicine* references *Users' guides* as a more detailed account of the whole programme (Straus et al. 2011: 8). Nevertheless, at times one text contains information not mentioned in the other. As a consequence, for the remainder of this book I refer to both *Users' guides* and *Evidence-based medicine* as the two primary sources of the details of EBM concepts and practice. I also draw primarily upon the most recent editions of the books, given that they reflect EBM in its present iteration, although

---

[1] Hereafter *Evidence-based medicine*.

[2] Sackett is considered by many to have been the original and most influential proponent of EBM in its current form.

[3] Hereafter *Users' guides*.

I refer to past editions to illustrate the evolution of basic concepts or note-worthy discrepancies.

2.1.2 **Defining EBM**

In *Evidence-based medicine*, Straus and colleagues do not define EBM, but write that it requires '. . . the integration of the best research evidence[4] with our clinical expertise[5] and our patient's unique values[6] and circumstances'[7] (2011: 1). Similarly, *Users' guides* states that 'evidence-based clinical practice requires integration of individual clinical expertise and patient preferences with the best available external clinical evidence from systematic research and consideration of available resources' (Guyatt et al. 2008: 783). In this latter definition, the authors introduce the idea that consideration of costs is also part of evidence-based practice. Yet both texts are mainly devoted to the issues of how to find and understand research data, rather than to details about clinical expertise, patient preferences, or consideration of available resources. Furthermore, the texts offer little explanation of what is meant by integration of these three spheres, or explain how integration works when there are conflicts between evidence, expertise, and values.

2.1.3 **Primacy of Evidence**

In describing the original idea behind EBM, *Users' guides* emphasizes the primacy of evidence, promoting '. . . an attitude of "enlightened scepticism" toward the application of diagnostic, therapeutic, and prognostic technologies in [the day-to-day management of patients]. . . . The goal is to be aware of the evidence on which one's practice is based, the soundness of the evidence, and the strength of inference the evidence permits' (Guyatt et al. 2008: xxi). In writing

---

[4] Best research evidences is defined as '. . . clinically relevant research, sometimes from the basic sciences of medicine, but especially from patient-centred clinical research into the accuracy and precision of diagnostic tests (including the clinical examination), the power of prognostic markers, and the efficacy and safety of therapeutic, rehabilitative, and preventive strategies' (Straus et al. 2011: 1).

[5] Clinical expertise is defined as '. . . the ability to use our clinical skills and past experience to rapidly identify each patient's unique health state and diagnosis, their individual risks and benefits of potential interventions, and their personal values and expectations' (Straus et al. 2011: 1).

[6] Patient values are defined as '. . . the unique preferences, concerns and expectations each patient brings to a clinical encounter and which must be integrated into clinical decisions if they are to serve the patient' (Straus et al. 2011: 1).

[7] Patient circumstances are defined as '. . . their individual clinical state and the clinical setting' (Straus et al. 2011: 1).

about the present edition of *Users' guides*, the authors say: 'the objective of this book is to help you make efficient use of the published literature in guiding your patient care' (Guyatt et al. 2008: 4).

Therefore, even in the most recent descriptions of EBM there remains some ambiguity about whether practising EBM involves combining evidence, clinical expertise, and patients' values in individual patient encounters, or whether EBM is primarily focused on applying research data extracted from the medical literature directly to individual clinical decision-making. In order to practise EBM the practitioner needs to know where the emphasis is placed: is it on evidence as the most important factor or is evidence one of several equally important factors?

2.1.4 Empirical Observation

The centrepiece of EBM is the term 'evidence', since it is upon evidence that medicine is to be based. *Users' guides* defines 'potential evidence' as 'any empirical observation' (Guyatt et al. 2008: 10). *Evidence-based medicine* does not define evidence but does provide the following description of best research evidence:

> . . . clinically relevant research, sometimes from the basic science of medicine, but especially from patient-centred clinical research into the accuracy and precision of diagnostic tests (including the clinical examination), the power of prognostic markers, and the efficacy and safety of therapeutic, rehabilitative, and preventive regimens.
>
> (Straus et al. 2011: 1)

The 2005 edition offered a similar definition, different only in two words. In that edition, best research evidence was defined as:

> . . . valid [now deleted] and clinically relevant research, often [now reads 'sometimes'] from the basic science of medicine, but especially from patient-centred clinical research into the accuracy and precision of diagnostic tests (including the clinical examination), the power of prognostic markers, and the efficacy and safety of therapeutic, rehabilitative, and preventive regimens.
>
> (Straus et al. 2005: 1)

Why did the authors choose to de-emphasize validity and research from the basic science of medicine? They do not contrast the present definition with the earlier one, so this is unknown.

2.1.5 Hierarchy of Evidence

The phrase 'clinically relevant research' is expounded further by the evidence hierarchy. The hierarchy is a ranking of research methods, of which the basic claim is that certain research methods are more likely than others to yield accurate data and therefore truthful conclusions about the topic being researched. The idea behind the hierarchy is to direct clinicians, who are consulting the medical literature on a specific clinical question, to studies that use the highest-ranked methods. This hierarchy of methods becomes a hierarchy of evidence because data produced by higher-ranked methods supplant data produced by lower-ranked methods on the grounds that the methods used to generate them are, a priori, superior in generating truthful information.

Clinicians are supposed to base their clinical decision-making on the highest-ranked data available. How data generated by methods not listed on the hierarchy should be considered is not specified. For example, *Users' guides* does include a chapter on qualitative research methods but this chapter notes that qualitative research in the health care context focuses on 'social and interpreted phenomena' rather than quantifiable or natural ones. It further states that these methods do not aim to 'test and evaluate' and that 'a qualitative study will not tell you whether an intervention achieved benefit (a randomized trial is best for that question)' (Guyatt et al. 2008: 344).

These statements imply that unlisted methods are unlisted because they cannot provide data that are needed to answer the questions of greatest importance within EBM: questions of diagnosis, prognosis, treatment, and harm. Therefore, the reader might infer that what the authors mean by evidence for clinical decision-making on any of these four domains is quite straightforwardly the data produced by the methods named in the hierarchy.

2.1.6 **Best Evidence**

Best research evidence is data derived from research methods at the top of the hierarchy. Clinicians should seek out data produced by the highest-ranked methods possible, working their way down the hierarchy until they are able to retrieve data on the clinical question of interest. The authors note that different domains have different hierarchies of methods. For example, there is a different hierarchy of research methods against which to judge studies which evaluate the sensitivity and specificity of diagnostic tests, compared to the hierarchy of methods for testing new treatments. This book focuses primarily on the hierarchy of evidence for treatment interventions, since most clinical research in psychiatry is done to evaluate treatments rather than to evaluate diagnostic tests or to assess prognosis.

Users' guides provides the following ranking of research methods that an evidence-based practitioner should use in order to evaluate articles about new treatments:

> N-of-1 randomized trials[8]
> Systematic reviews[9] of randomized trials
> Single randomized trial
> Systematic review of observational studies addressing patient-important outcomes
> Single observational study addressing patient-important outcomes
> Physiologic studies
> Unsystematic clinical observations[10]

(Guyatt et al. 2008: 11)

Evidence-based medicine does not provide a hierarchy for studies of treatments or other interventions; however, the text describes the research methods against which published studies should be judged. For example, an individual study of a new treatment that is double-blind,[11] randomized,[12] and controlled would be of the highest standard; trials that included some, but not all, of these criteria would fall somewhat below the standard, and so forth. Over the years, a plethora of EBM sources have emerged, sometimes listing hierarchies that differed from the one offered by *Users' guides* (Upshur 2003). This raises the question of which version of the hierarchy individual practitioners should use.

----

[8] An n-of-1 randomized trial is 'an experiment designed to determine the effect of an intervention or exposure on a single study participant. In one n-of-1 design, the patient undergoes pairs of treatment periods organized so that 1 period involves the use of the experimental treatment and 1 period involves the use of an alternate treatment or placebo. The patient and clinician are blinded if possible, and outcomes are monitored. Treatment periods are replicated until the clinician and patient are convinced that the treatments are definitely different or definitely not different' (Guyatt et al. 2008: 792).

[9] A systematic review is 'a summary of the clinical literature that uses explicit methods to perform a comprehensive literature search and critical appraisal of individual studies and that may use appropriate statistical techniques to combine these valid studies when appropriate. The statistical technique for pooling studies is called a meta-analysis' (Straus et al. 2011: 273).

[10] New versions of the hierarchy are being developed. For example, see: <http://www.cebm. net/index.aspx?o=1025> (accessed 26 January 2014).

[11] Double-blind means that neither the investigator nor the study participant know whether they have been assigned to the experimental group or the control group.

[12] Randomized means that study participants are allocated randomly to either the study group or the control group.

2.1.7 **The GRADE System**

In recent years, some leading EBM authors have been part of a working group trying to develop a single ranking system that assesses the quality of a body of evidence (GRADE). Unlike the hierarchy, this system does not automatically assign highest status to a study based solely on its type. For example, even though randomized controlled trials (RCTs) are near the top of the hierarchy, given certain methodological conditions the quality of a specific trial may be low.

The GRADE system is designed to enable authors or organizations to take these types of differences into consideration when examining the literature on a specific topic or when making clinical recommendations on a topic. The authors hope that the many organizations such as professional associations and health technology assessment bodies charged with the tasks of assessing the medical literature on specific topics and issuing practice guidelines or recommendations will adopt their particular system, which they believe will facilitate communication and comparison.

2.1.8 **Further Specifications**

In the phrase 'evidence-based medicine', 'evidence-based' is used as an adjective, implying that medicine represents something distinct from EBM. *Users' guides* contrasts EBM with 'the traditional paradigm of medical practice', stating that 'EBM places lower value' on unsystematic clinical experience, pathophysiologic rationale, and authority' (Guyatt et al. 2008: 10). This statement implies that, prior to EBM, these sources of information predominated in medicine. The 2002 edition of *Users' guides* offered a stronger claim, saying that clinical experience and pathophysiologic rationale (as well as intuition—which is not mentioned in the 2008 edition) were insufficient grounds for clinical decision-making, as opposed to merely being of lower value (Guyatt et al. 2002: 4).

Likewise, *Evidence-based medicine* does not formally define medicine, but in its preface describes how each author became acquainted with the ideas behind EBM, and contrasts these ideas with their experiences of medicine (pre-EBM or non-EBM medicine). For one author, being challenged to 'provide evidence to support her management plans for each patient' is contrasted with situations where 'the management plan was learned by rote and was based on whatever the current consultant favored' (Straus et al. 2011: xiii). For another author, when asking a lecturer for the evidence in support of theories he was presenting, the lecturer replied that '. . . there wasn't any good evidence, and that he didn't believe the theories, but he had been asked by the head of the department "to give the talk"' (Straus et al. 2011: xiv). *Evidence-based medicine* also contrasts authoritative advice (evidence-based) with authoritarian advice (opinion-based) (Straus et al. 2011: 4). These characterizations suggest that medicine involves the uncritical acceptance of information, determined primarily by power relations and local predispositions.

2.1.9 Shift of Definition

The shifts in definitions between editions are noteworthy because they suggest that EBM has softened its claims. For example, according to *Users' guides*, unsystematic clinical observation and pathophysiologic rationale are no longer insufficient grounds for clinical decisions as had been the case in the 2002 edition, but are merely of lower value. However, the texts do not specify when and how these lower-value elements should operate. Further, in defining best research evidence, *Evidence-based medicine* deletes the term 'valid' in describing 'clinically relevant research', suggesting that perhaps research that is clinically relevant may not always meet EBM's concept of validity. How one weighs relevance against validity when these aspects are in conflict is also not specified. *Users' guides* notes that the hierarchy of evidence is 'not absolute' (Guyatt et al. 2008: 12), and goes on to say that in certain circumstances (related to strength of study design), lower-ranked sources may provide stronger evidence than higher-ranked sources, although it acknowledges that knowing when this is the case is challenging.

In earlier iterations of EBM, the authors worried that individual clinical observation and individual judgements about relevance or validity of research could not be trusted, hence the need for strict rules about what could be allowed as the basis of clinical decisions. As this position softens and the rules become less strict, EBM must specify how and when individual interpretation is allowed. However, the texts do not provide such specification; therefore, the mechanics of how to practise EBM under the revised definitions are somewhat less clear compared to earlier editions of the texts. Furthermore, without such specification the reader might wonder how this is substantively different from what preceded EBM.

2.1.10 Positivism and Consequentialism

Underlying these definitions, both texts make allusions to key philosophical commitments including positivism and consequentialism. Positivism, a philosophical movement dominant between the 1920s and 1950s, had various aims, one of which was to detail a scientific basis for philosophy. Its leading proponents posited (among other things) that only empirically verifiable statements could have meaning and thus count towards knowledge. For example, a statement such as 'the patient is in the waiting room' counted as possible knowledge, whereas a statement such as 'this article is good' was meaningless because it was not straightforwardly veri-fiable or falsifiable.

Ultimately, positivism was defeated as an epistemological position because of the difficulty in elucidating the specifics of a principle of verification. Yet elements of positivism remain deeply influential in contemporary medicine and even more so in EBM. The notion that true knowledge must be verifi-able or falsifiable using certain empirical methods is evident in what EBM includes as evidence and the allowable ways to obtain evidence. The more difficult it is to verify data, the more these very data are marginalized or even dismissed altogether by EBM. For example, feelings that arise in the clini-cian during a clinical encounter may be diagnostically informative, offering information as to a patient's state of mind, intentions, fears, and so on, yet these are difficult to verify, and such sources of knowledge do not appear on the evidence hierarchy for diagnostics. EBM texts do not explicitly state that these sources of data should be rejected, but because they devote no text to the details of such data, it stands to reason that they are perceived as less important than the results of certain types of research that receive hundreds of pages of discussion.

Consequentialism is the ethical theory stating that the moral value of an act is found in its consequences rather than in the actor or the action itself. Utilitarianism is a form of consequentialism in which moral value is located in the amount of utility (often defined as happiness or pleasure) or disutility resulting from an action. These theories form the ethical backbone of EBM, and its commitment to them is evident in its emphasis on doing more good than harm and in its specific use of the language of utility and disutility (Guyatt et al. 2008: 604; Straus et al. 2011: 97).

In fact, EBM links positivism and utilitarianism by associating a failure to use what can be verified about medical interventions with a failure to offer patients the highest utility—in the form of improved health outcomes. It seems that EBM's primary purpose, therefore, is to improve patients' health outcomes. It is unclear how other ethical considerations—such as duties to tell patients the truth or to work in their interest—factor into EBM's vision of practice. Are these other considerations understood to be part of EBM or part of medical practice into which EBM then inserts itself? These ques-tions are central to the investigation of the ethics of EBM in subsequent chapters.

The two key EBM textbooks provide little further explanation of EBM's core concepts. The remainder of both texts is devoted to understanding the technical details of certain types of study design and data analytic techniques. Haynes, a leading EBM originator, has pointed out that some central conceptual and ethical questions remain unaddressed by EBM and require attention (2002). These include questions of how to resolve conflicts between evidence and of whether patients who receive evidence-based practice actually do achieve better health—and if they do, how to ensure that benefits are distributed justly. Some of these questions are relevant to the present analysis of the ethics of EBM and are discussed more fully in other chapters. But before exploring such issues, the rest of this chapter summarizes how EBM is applied to clinical practice—in other words, how it actually works—as described in the EBM texts, *Evidence-based medicine* and *Users' guides*.

2.2 **The Practice of EBM**

EBM is a complex concept, proposing multiple things at once. First, it promotes a specific method for formulating what it considers to be the most important kinds of clinical questions arising in patient care, known as the PICO format.[13] Once the questions are formulated this way, EBM suggests resources that reference the kinds of research that can answer these questions. Second, EBM provides criteria by which to judge the capacity of research studies to yield truthful answers to these questions (a process called critical appraisal). The evidence hierarchy ranks research methods according to those that are most to least valid, according to its definition of what counts as validity in clinical research. Finally, EBM also suggests a method of making clinical decisions, particularly those concerning whether to use specific diagnostic tests and prescribe specific treatments (a process called decision analysis).

In *Evidence-based medicine*, practising EBM is described as a five-step process (see Box 2.1).

Evidence-based medicine explains that there are three ways to practise EBM: doing mode, using mode, or replicating mode (Straus et al. 2011: 3). The authors believe that (evidence-based) practitioners will shift between modes depending on the clinical problem at hand and their own level of knowledge. Doing mode involves carrying out all steps oneself. Using mode involves omitting step 3 by relying on pre-appraised sources in which someone else has critically appraised the original research studies. Replicating

---

[13] PICO is a way of posing clinical questions in which P stands for patient, population, predicament, or problem; I stands for intervention; C stands for a comparator; and O stands for an outcome of interest: for example, in patients with panic disorder, does sertraline reduce the frequency of panic attacks compared to placebo?

Box 2.1 The Five Steps of EBM

Step 1—converting the need for information (about prevention, diagnosis, prognosis, therapy, causation etc.) into an answerable question

Step 2—tracking down the best evidence with which to answer that question

Step 3—critically appraising that evidence for its validity (closeness to the truth), impact (size of the effect) and applicability (usefulness in our clinical practice)

Step 4—integrating the critical appraisal with our clinical expertise and with our patient's unique biology, values and circumstances

Step 5—evaluating our effectiveness and efficiency in executing steps 1—4 and seeking ways to improve them both for the next time

Data from Straus, S. E., Richardson, W. S., Glasziou, P., and Haynes, R. B., eds, Evidence-based medicine: how to practice and teach EBM, 4th ed., p. 3, Elsevier Churchill Livingstone, Edinburgh, 2011.

mode involves omitting steps 2 and 3 and following the decisions of 'respected opinion leaders'. The text goes on to say that these opinions may turn out to not be evidence-based at all, but that this too counts as evidence-based practice because the authors note that each mode requires the practitioner to integrate (step 4). Integration, at least according to the authors of *Evidence-based medicine*, is the sine qua non of EBM. The text of *Users' guides* covers similar material without laying out the five steps. The description in the following sections provides an overview of the five steps of evidence-based practice and draws on both texts.

2.2.1 Step 1—Asking Answerable Questions

In *Evidence-based medicine*, asking answerable questions refers to constructing content-orientated questions about specific medical topics. This step groups most questions into two types: background and foreground. Background questions ask for general knowledge about disorders, tests, treatments, or other aspects of health care and take the following form: 1) a question root with a verb, and 2) an aspect of condition or thing of interest. Foreground questions have four components, for which PICO can be used as a mnemonic device: P for the patient, population, predicament, or problem; I for the intervention, exposure, test, or other agent; C for the comparison intervention, exposure test, etc. (if relevant); and O for the outcomes of clinical importance, including time when relevant (Straus et al. 2011: 15–16). An example of a background question is: 'What causes panic disorder?' An example of a foreground question is: 'In patients with panic disorder, does sertraline reduce the frequency of panic attacks compared to placebo?'

Users' guides provides a very similar discussion of question formulation in the chapter entitled 'Finding the evidence', using the same terminology (background and foreground questions) and the same structures for these types of questions. In addition, this text states that there are five fundamental types of clinical questions, which involve therapy, harm, differential diagnosis, diagnosis, and prognosis (Guyatt et al. 2008: 20). *Evidence-based medicine* includes a longer list of clinical questions, including those relating to 'clinical findings, etiology/risk, clinical manifestations of disease, differential diagnosis, diagnostic tests, prognosis, therapy, prevention, experience and meaning, and improvement' (Straus et al. 2011: 18).

Evidence-based medicine implies that the main advantage of the PICO format is that it conforms, to the greatest extent, to the ways that research questions in medical studies are asked and indexed by standard medical databases such as Medline and EMBASE. It is in this sense that asking answerable questions is so important, because there must be potential to find answers in the medical research literature. Why? *Evidence-based medicine* states: 'when our questions get answered, our knowledge grows, our curiosity is reinforced, our cognitive resonance is restored, and we can become better, faster, and happier clinicians' (Straus et al. 2011: 21). How should the clinician handle questions that are not amenable to the PICO format, questions that clinical researchers choose not to address, or questions that are difficult to answer or are unanswerable? These issues are not discussed.

2.2.2 **Step 2—Finding Evidence**

Finding evidence, according to *Evidence-based medicine,* should be done in accordance with the '6S hierarchy', which ranks sources of information. These sources, from highest to lowest, include systems, summaries, synopses of syntheses, syntheses, synopses of studies, and studies (Straus et al. 2011: 33–9).

Systems are considered to be the ideal but not yet available. This category refers to computerized decision support systems, which are computer programs that summarize the research data about the diagnosis, prognosis, and treatment of a clinical problem, and ideally link to patients' electronic medical records, prompting the clinician about data relevant to that patient's clinical care. Properly designed, these programs should be automatically updated when new data regarding problems are available. In practice, the electronic health record itself will prompt clinicians into evidence-based interventions: for example, the support system will prompt clinicians treating a patient with major depression to be aware of the treatments with the highest possible ratings according to the evidence hierarchy.

Summaries include evidence-based textbooks or searchable online resources that organize and summarize topics and the evidence relating to those topics, such as *UpToDate*. Synopses of syntheses are publications that select and, using a prescribed (structured) format, summarize high-quality systematic review studies, where quality is defined according to how closely the included studies adhere to the principles of EBM criteria. The quality is rated by the synopses' authors. EBM's authors describe this as 'pre-appraised' evidence, meaning that step 3 (critical appraisal) has already been carried out; the job of the clinician is simply to locate these sources. Syntheses are databases of systematic reviews of the research studies on a specific topic selected by the authors and judged according to explicit criteria. The best known of these is the Cochrane Database of Systematic Reviews. Synopses of studies are similar to synopses of syntheses, except that they only summarize one study rather than groups of studies. An example of a psychiatry-specific source of synopses is the journal *Evidence-Based Mental Health*, whose entire content is a series of structured summaries of research papers that have been selected because they are of the highest methodological quality, according to EBM's methodology criteria. The studies category refers to original studies as published in academic journals.

Users' guides mentions a '4S strategy' (systems, synopses, summaries, and studies), using slightly different definitions from *Evidence-based medicine*. Systems are again at the top, but are defined in the way that *Evidence-based medicine* defines summaries. Synopses are defined in the same manner. Ranked next are summaries, which are defined as *Evidence-based medicine* defines syntheses. Original studies are ranked last.

Critically appraising individual studies was the hallmark of the EBM approach in its beginning, but after 20 years of evolution its texts now rate original studies lowest as sources of evidence. *Users' guides* notes that original studies require individual clinicians to engage in critical appraisal themselves, while in all the higher-ranked sources this step has been done already. Note that this approach to finding evidence applies to foreground questions: *Users' guides* and *Evidence-based medicine* state that background questions are likely to be best answered by medical textbooks (Guyatt et al. 2008: 18; Straus et al. 2011: 30–1).

An issue worth noting is the absolute necessity of ready-at-hand internet access in the workplace, as well as paid subscriptions to pre-appraised resources and academic journals in order to practise EBM. Furthermore, several EBM authors are involved in the production of these resources. For example, a source highly recommended by both texts – the *ACP Journal Club* – has, as its editor, an individual who is also an author of *Evidence-Based Medicine* and a contributor to the *Users' Guides*. As a result, these authors are in a type of conflict of interest in promoting these for-profit resources, inasmuch as they have a duty to the millions of colleagues who read their work to adopt a disinterested stance, while on the other hand they stand to benefit from the sale of EBM products (Upshur et al. 2006).

2.2.3 Steps 3 and 4—Critical Appraisal and Integration

In *Evidence-based medicine* steps 3 (critical appraisal) and 4 (integration) are discussed together, while in *Users' guides* these steps are not described as such. *Users' guides* does, however, outline similar content to that found in the descriptions of steps 3 and 4 in *Evidence-based medicine*.

The process of critical appraisal does not begin with an analysis of the original data presented in a study. Instead, both texts lay out general criteria for assessing the quality of research studies. There are also specific criteria depending on whether a study is evaluating a diagnostic test, the prognosis of a condition, or the effectiveness or harmfulness of an intervention. I have not discussed each set of rules in detail. Instead, I focus on the rules that are applicable to all types of studies with specific attention to the rules governing therapy, as these are the rules most applicable to psychiatry where most of the existing evidence is generated through studies of treatments.

In reviewing any type of study, readers are told, they should ask three fundamental questions: 1) Are the results valid? 2) What are the results (what is the size of the effect)? and 3) How can I apply these results to patient care (or to a specific patient)? (Guyatt et al. 2008: 6). For the authors of *Evidence-based medicine* these questions comprise step 3 (critical appraisal), while the last question, determining applicability, is also related to step 4 (integration): 'to apply evidence, we need to integrate the evidence with our clinical experience and expertise, and with our patient's values and preferences' (Straus et al. 2011: 88).

Users' guides does not describe integration as a term, but does discuss how to apply research results to patient care. It also introduces another term—incorporation—as in 'EBM requires the incorporation of patients' values and preferences into decision making' (Guyatt et al. 2008: 644). *Evidence-based medicine* also uses the term incorporation, but specifically to describe the process of assigning a numerical value to a patient's preference and combining that quantitatively with other quantitative values such as the number needed to treat (NNT).[14] Let us now look at each of the three questions involved in steps 3 and 4.

2.2.3.1 Are the Results Valid?

To determine a study's validity is to assess its 'closeness to the truth' (Straus et al. 2011: 3). In order to make this determination, the reader must assess a study's design. According to both texts, certain designs are associated, inherently, with greater validity because they minimize bias. Bias is a '. . . systematic deviation from the underlying truth because of a feature of the design or conduct of a research study' (Guyatt et al. 2008: 771). While there are specific criteria for validity that apply to different types of studies depending on whether the study evaluates a treatment, a diagnostic test, prognosis of a condition, or harm caused, *Evidence-based medicine*'s authors offer a general strategy for thinking about the considerations of validity applicable to any type of study. These include considering: 1) how the participants were identified and selected and whether they were fairly assigned to intervention or control; 2) whether the participants were treated the same throughout the study, and 3) whether the outcomes were measured objectively and whether the analysis was conducted properly (Straus et al., 2011: 63). For studies of treatment, RCTs—preferably those that are double-blinded—are considered to yield results closest to the truth. In addition, the study groups have to be prognostically similar and their follow-up has to be sufficiently long. Apart from receiving different experimental treatments, groups should be treated equally. The rules for assessing validity also include aspects of data analysis: participants should be analysed as belonging to the groups in which they started, regardless of what actually happened in the course of the study (intention-to-treat analysis).

2.2.3.2 What are the Results (What is the Size of the Effect)?

The size of a study's effect refers to the magnitude of difference made by an intervention and is determined by the absolute change attributable to the intervention under study. This change can be reported using a variety of numerical representations. Readers are encouraged to seek out translations of the reported data into clinically meaningful numbers such as the NNT (the inverse of the absolute risk reduction). Precision of effect is also critical to assessing

---

[14] The NNT is '. . . the number of patients who need to be treated during a specific period of time to achieve 1 additional good outcome'. Similarly, the NNH (number needed to harm) is '. . . the number of patients who, if they received the experimental intervention, would lead to 1 additional patient harmed during a specific period' (Guyatt et al. 2008: 793).

importance. The texts recommend the use of confidence intervals—the statistically plausible ranges for specific values—to determine precision.

2.2.3.3 How can I Apply these Results to Patient Care (or to a Specific Patient)?

There are four components to this question. Application of research data is the result of addressing each of the four components. Integration of evidence with clinical expertise is the result of addressing the first three components, while integration of evidence with patients' values and preferences is the process of answering the fourth component (see Figure 2.1).

The first component is the assessment of whether one's patients are sufficiently biologically and sociodemographically similar to those who participated in the study under review that the results can be generalized to them. *Evidence-based medicine* tells us that whether the similarity makes sense is determined by clinical expertise. The second component concerns feasibility, which is specifically discussed in terms of affordability (will someone—the patient, an insurer, the health system—be able to pay for it?) and availability (Straus et al. 2011: 90). The third component asks what are the potential benefits and harms of the intervention. Benefits and harms are to be represented numerically by adjusting the NNT and NNH to take into consideration increased or decreased risk given the patient's health status, compared to study participants in the trial under consideration. This adjustment is made by applying prognostic data of groups more similar to the patient, such as data from other studies or from a similar subgroup in the study being appraised. The fourth component asks what the patient's values and expectations are with respect to the intervention and the outcome targeted.

Both texts lay out quantitative methods of eliciting and ranking patient preferences for the health outcomes under discussion as a way of integrating or incorporating patients' values (in this context the terms integration

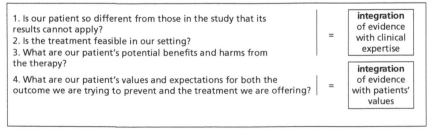

Fig. 2.1 Application of evidence to an individual patient. Data from Straus, S. E., Richardson, W. S., Glasziou, P., and Haynes, R. B., eds, Evidence-based medicine: How to practice and teach EBM, 4th ed., Elsevier Churchill Livingstone, Edinburgh, 2011.

and incorporation are used interchangeably). First, one should compute the likelihood of being helped or harmed (LHH), a ratio of the NNT to the NNH that can be adjusted to take into account an individual patient's risk factors. The LHH can then be manipulated further to reflect the patient's numerical tradeoff of benefits versus harms of an intervention (e.g. by assigning numerical values to the desirability or undesirability of health outcomes). This method attempts to ensure that patients' preferences guide decision-making. Both texts state that the ideal method for incorporating patients' values is a process called 'clinical decision analysis', in which all relevant outcomes of an intervention are compared numerically, according to the probabilities of these events and the utility (represented numerically from 0 to 1) the patient associates with them. Probability and utility are multiplied and the option and the right treatment decision would then be the one leading to the highest utility. *Evidence-based medicine* laments the fact that decision analysis takes too much time to be feasible. Neither text explains where other values—those of clinicians, families, institutions, or society—fit into this picture or how to handle situations in which patients' values are in conflict with other considerations such as cost, availability, and institutional structures (e.g. waiting lists, inclusion/exclusion criteria).

2.2.4 **Step 5—Self-evaluation**

Self-evaluation of EBM practice involves determining how well one is adhering to the instructions and tasks of the first four steps. The self-evaluation questions entailed by each of these steps are listed in Table 2.1.

Unlike the first three steps, the self-evaluation questions for step 4 do not map fully onto the content of the step as described in the text. Recall that step 4 was to integrate one's critical appraisal with our clinical expertise and with our patient's unique biology, values, and circumstances. However, the questions do not refer to the point at which patients and clinicians actually discuss values. Even in the text that accompanies the step 4 self-evaluation questions under the heading, 'Evaluating our performance in integrating evidence and patients' values' (Straus ct al. 2011: 206–9), values are not actually mentioned. Do the authors believe that integrating patients' values cannot be evaluated? This is not explained.

Although changing practice behaviour is not one of the five steps, the authors of *Evidence-based medicine* add this final element to self-evaluation (Table 2.2).

While this section does not reflect the extensive detail provided in these texts about the methods for executing the five steps, it is noteworthy that the remaining detail is largely technical and invites the reader to master the concepts through examples and practical exercises. The practice of EBM

Table 2.1 The self-evaluation questions associated with the first four steps of evidence-based practice

The steps of evidence-based practice	Self-evaluation questions for each step
Step 1: asking answerable questions	1. Am I asking any clinical questions at all? 2. Am I asking focused questions? 3. Am I using a map to locate my knowledge gaps and articulate questions? 4. Can I get myself unstuck when asking questions? 5. Do I have a working method to save my questions for later answering?
Step 2: finding the best external evidence	1. Am I searching at all? 2. Do I know the best sources of current evidence for my clinical discipline? 3. Do I have easy access to the best evidence for my clinical discipline? 4. Am I becoming more efficient in my searching? 5. Am I using truncations, booleans, MeSH headings, thesaurus limiters, and intelligent free text when searching MEDLINE? 6. How do my searches compare with those of research librarians or other respected colleagues who have a passion for providing best current patient care?
Step 3: critically appraising the evidence for its validity and potential usefulness	1. Am I critically appraising external evidence at all? 2. Are the critical appraisal guides becoming easier for me to apply? 3. Am I becoming more accurate and efficient in applying some of the critical appraisal measures (such as likelihood ratios, NNTs and the like)? 4. Am I creating any appraisal summaries?
Step 4: integrating one's critical appraisal with our clinical expertise and with our patient's unique biology, values and circumstances	1. Am I integrating my critical appraisals into my practice at all? 2. Am I becoming more accurate and efficient in adjusting some of the critical appraisal measures to fit my individual patients (pre-test probabilities, NNT/f etc.)? 3. Can I explain (and resolve) disagreements about management decisions in terms of this integration?

Data from Straus, S. E., Richardson, W. S., Glasziou, P., and Haynes, R. B., eds, Evidence-based medicine: how to practice and teach EBM, 4th ed., Elsevier Churchill Livingstone, Edinburgh, 2011.

then, is no more than these five steps, at least according to these authoritative texts.

2.2.5 What is the Purpose of EBM?

In all these details about evidence-based practice, its primary purpose remains unclear. Both texts agree that 'evidence-based medicine is about solving clinical

Table 2.2 The self-evaluation questions associated with the final element

Final element of evidence-based practice	Self-evaluation questions
Changing practice behaviour	1. When evidence suggests a change in practice, am I identifying barriers and facilitators to this change? 2. Have I identified a strategy to implement this change, targeted to the barriers I've identified? 3. Have I carried out any check, such as audits of my diagnostic, therapeutic, or other EBM performance, including evidence use as well as impact on clinical outcomes? 4. Am I considering sustainability of this change?

Data from Straus, S. E., Richardson, W. S., Glasziou, P., and Haynes, R. B., eds, Evidence-based medicine: how to practice and teach EBM, 4th ed., pp. 206–9, Elsevier Churchill Livingstone, Edinburgh, 2011.

problems' (Guyatt et al. 2008: 10; Straus et al. 2011: 30) without specifying what kinds of solutions it aims to achieve. Nevertheless, there are various clues scattered throughout both texts. For example, the self-evaluation questions discussed in Section 2.2.4 suggest that the proper practice of EBM involves mastery of the techniques described in the individual steps (literature searching, analysing methods, manipulating the figures presented in studies, etc.) but this simply denotes that successful practice of EBM means understanding and executing the five steps. At another point in *Evidence-based medicine* (Straus et al. 2011: 5) the authors discuss briefly the various studies that have tried to evaluate EBM educational interventions. They state that these interventions have tried to produce a range of outcomes including changes in practitioners' knowledge and skills (of the five steps), and behaviour and attitudes (towards EBM). However, they also mention that EBM educational interventions have been evaluated to see whether they led to improved health outcomes. Similarly, the additional evaluative step focusing on 'changing practice behavior' also includes the question of whether EBM has led to an impact on clinical outcomes (see Table 2.2).

This discussion highlights two different goals of EBM: to effect changes in practitioners (their knowledge, skills, behaviour and attitudes) while at the same time improving patients' health outcomes. In both texts the authors cite the results of certain high-profile clinical trials, which demonstrated that the drugs under investigation, although thought to be effective, actually caused harm by doing the opposite of what they were thought to do (Guyatt et al.

2008: 120 and 134; Straus et al. 2011: 69 and 186). These examples support the idea that EBM's purpose is to improve the health of patients, particularly by demonstrating which interventions are useless or even harmful. Failure to adhere to EBM would be to continue to offer treatments that were potentially ineffective or harmful. Put this way, practising EBM is ethically necessary. Thus, this is a third goal of EBM: to offer more ethical practice in the sense of leading to better consequences for patients.

2.3 **Conceptual Clarification—Experts Define EBM**

In spite of the fact that there are entire books devoted to the description of EBM, the interviewees, many of whom had considerable expertise in the field, spoke at length about the challenges of trying to define and understand EBM and related concepts such as evidence. In this section, I look at how these experts became involved in EBM, how they define it, and then compare this with how EBM is defined in its authoritative texts. I identify and explore some key, unsettled issues that arise in trying to define EBM.

My interviewees became interested in EBM for a variety of reasons. Those who were EBM developers explained that EBM appealed to their desire to understand how and why medical decisions are made, and to have the tools to be able to challenge people's thinking and decision-making in a rational way.

> 1–2: '. . . up until then it was very much more of a traditional kind of educational approach, and it was whatever your staff physician told you this is what you did. And so really I found very empowering, that they were actually talking to us about getting skills so that we could actually be better consumers of the literature and understand what it was.'

> 1-6: '. . . what was appealing to me was to be a little bit more in depth and being able to assess the evidence by myself so I can resist and I can have arguments in my hands . . .'

Like EBM developers, mental health experts were interested, even concerned, about how clinical decisions are made. Their interest in EBM stemmed from the worry that clinical thinking in mental health was overly theoretically preoccupied.

> 2-6: '. . . as a resident sitting in grand rounds in child psychiatry when they were talking . . . somebody was presenting a case about eating disorder. And the person presenting the case was very much into family therapy and made the comment that, really, the driving motivation in this girl's psychopathology was the fact that she had a distant father and an over-involved mother. I said to myself: "That's what they say about everybody regardless of what the problem is." So I thought to myself: "What I'm being taught in terms of etiologic factors is not very discriminatory. It doesn't

discriminate among different sorts of problems." So that was what really made me, as a resident, begin to think about how we think about etiologic factors in psychopathology. And then I did a degree in clinical epidemiology. So I have a master's degree in clinical epidemiology where I learned about critical appraisal and I've always been a strong proponent of trying to introduce more critical appraisal into practice.'

Many participants encountered EBM directly through their work as researchers, where it was particularly important to understand concepts such as evidence.

2-10: 'I didn't become interested in EBM as such, but in research and science and concepts of psychiatry. And I did research and doing research means coming across the term as a concept, and the idea and the objectivity of evidence...'

Meanwhile, the philosophers/bioethicists had become interested in EBM for a wider variety of reasons. For some, an academic focus on clinical ethics was an entrée to this topic.

3-2: '... that's why I became more and more interested in evidence-based medicine or cost-effective analysis because I had a long-term interest in resource allocation, justice issues in health care.'

3-9: 'I became quite interested in decisions under uncertainty. I mean, if you were my physician, at what point is it appropriate for you to make a prescribing decision? For example, based on a meta-analysis as opposed to a randomized trial . . . That raised the ethical issues related to informed consent. . .'

Others became engaged with conceptual and philosophical issues posed by EBM.

3-5: '... it also looked like a very interesting area for me to think about in the philosophy of medicine. What's the foundation of medical knowledge? Is there such a thing as a clinical science or is medicine simply applications of biochemistry, pharmacology, physiology, and so on, that medicine doesn't have its own science? So I got interested in the idea of evidence-based medicine as an attempt to make a free-standing science of medicine with its own rules, its own laws, its own theory of causation, its own methodology for securing facts and so on.'

3-7: '... my real connection is from the side of logic and critical thinking.'

3-13: '... as a philosopher, of course, hearing the term "evidence" my ears prick up and I started to get really interested in what kinds of epistemological questions were relevant to EBM and that weren't being considered by the people who had developed it. My interest in the ethical aspects of EBM actually sort of comes through the epistemological aspect so, rather than taking maybe a more traditional approach in terms of moral theories, I'm interested in the ethical issues that arise when we think about evidence in a certain way or we choose to take certain epistemological approaches to medicine.'

This brief introduction to the respondents illustrates that EBM, the application of epidemiological principles to clinical practice, is an entry point for reflection from various disciplinary perspectives. In particular, EBM has attracted a great deal of attention from the fields of philosophy and ethics.

2.3.1 **What is EBM?**

There was general agreement among EBM developers about how to define EBM. Most respondents described EBM as a link between research knowledge and clinical practice. According to this framing, the terms 'knowledge' and 'evidence' refer to the same thing. It is part of evidence-based practice to be able to tell the difference between strong and weak evidence for whatever intervention is being considered in a given clinical situation. Group 1 participants believed that three common but erroneous perceptions exist about EBM: 1) that only RCT data count as evidence; 2) that all clinical decisions require RCT data to support them; and 3) that clinicians cannot responsibly offer interventions that had not been researched by RCTs. They resisted this characterization of EBM as an RCTs-or-nothing mentality. Instead, these participants focused on EBM as the generation and use of all types of research data (evidence) in combination with an awareness of patients' values in clinical decision-making.

> 1-2: '. . . so it's really about bringing the evidence, the best available evidence and a lot of times people think there is only one type of evidence, but it's really the best available evidence that we have that's out there with our clinical expertise and with our patient values, and it's really to me it's bringing those three pieces together.'

> 1-6: '. . . what EBM says among other things, is you need to know the evidence, and it also says that you should be able to assess the validity of this evidence or how to phrase it differently, the hierarchy of this evidence—the difference of different levels of believability, and by that I mean how trusting we are in estimates of effects of different interventions. So that is the first pillar of evidence-based medicine. Using the best available evidence, being able to distinguish between different quality of evidence, and recognizing also that evidence doesn't make the decision for you and that you need to know values and preferences of individual patients.'

2.3.2 **Convergences and Divergences**

In general, there was a convergence of views between the EBM developers on the formal definition of EBM, yet the question of what it means to be an evidence-based practitioner generated a greater variety of responses. For example, some respondents commented that critical appraisal skills (step 3 of EBM) could only be achieved through graduate-level training and/or intensive mentoring.

> 1-8: '. . .before I got into the master's programme, I took a 12-session course "how to look at the literature" . . . I did this as a resident. And at the end I thought: "Oh good, now I'll be able to read the literature." I started to read the methods and results,

couldn't do it. Gave up . . . 12 sessions of an hour and a half each were not enough to allow me to read the literature. And, in fact, I remember the way the programme was structured then, I did one course during the summer and then I did a statistics course and a "how to design an RCT" course in the autumn. And I remember it was about October that I started saying: "Hey, I can read methods and results now." That is what it took.'

3-10: 'I mean to me, being an EBM practitioner seems to carry with it a specific skill set that really, I don't know that you necessarily need an MPH [Master of Public Health] or a Master of Science of Epi [epidemiology] to do it, but more and more it seems like you do. As the analyses get more and more complex in a lot of this clinical research it takes somebody with a fairly developed skill set to interpret. . .'

Others believed that the practice of EBM involves a set of skills that have to be taught and fostered early on, but this could be done during clinical training. For clinicians who were already in practice, continuing education courses and practice could be sufficient to learn critical appraisal skills. However, some participants noted that one might also require a basic, pre-existing temperament or attitude in order to want to learn and use these skills in practice. As such, they feared the majority of practitioners would never learn theses skills in depth because they lacked either interest or at least aptitude.

Finally, some offered the view that a clinician who consults pre-appraised sources of evidence but never engages in critical appraisal herself could legitimately count herself as an evidence-based practitioner.

1-6: 'I would say the evidence-based practitioner is a person who knows which place, which textbook, which other practitioner, which clinical teacher behaves according to those principles and I do not think this person would necessarily need to go into details behind the final statements [contained in evidence-based resources].'

These views help to shed light on what EBM is by considering what an EBM practitioner is. Although developers of EBM agree on the formal definition of EBM as a tripartite structure that involves integrating best available evidence with clinical expertise and patients' values, they differed from one another considerably about what kind of knowledge and/or training is required to be able to do this. This ranged from formal graduate degrees in clinical epidemiology (in addition to undergraduate and postgraduate clinical training), to intensive training during the postgraduate years, to continuing medical education, and to simply learning how to identify which sources were and were not evidence-based. As one participant pointed out, in the absence of knowing what specific skill set was required to be an evidence-based practitioner, it is difficult to determine who would qualify and, therefore, what evidence-based practice really is.

2.3.3 **Humpty Dumpty**

The philosopher/bioethicists repeatedly raised the idea that EBM had many meanings and it was difficult to choose one because there were various accounts and it depended who one asked and which sources one privileged.

> 3-10: '. . . I keep finding myself thinking of Humpty Dumpty when he says, "A word means whatever I want it to mean, no more and no less", and that's what evidence-based medicine often is.'

These participants argued that this variability in the definition might reflect an evolution in the concept of EBM, whether as a result of a natural process of improvement or as a way of deflecting criticisms of the original formulation. One participant offered a more radical interpretation, suggesting that EBM is a catchphrase whose substantive meaning is intentionally unclear so as to give power to those who controlled it.

> 3-3: 'The emotive concept underlying EBM is in fact primary, and the descriptive concept we can then decide that later. So what's happening is you've got a group of people who are taking control of a professional area, claiming ownership of it by claiming ownership of the key persuasive terminology in that area. You make the term "evidence" yours, then you can decide at a later date what counts as evidence. You've claimed the authority to determine what's good and bad in that area, what ought to happen and what ought not to happen, what people have a warrant to do and what they don't have a warrant to do. So it struck me that evidence-based medicine really was a movement that . . . when it got going . . . its power was based on the seductiveness of the terminology.'

2.3.4 **Bureaucratic Tool**

Another interviewee took an equally dim view, seeing EBM primarily as a bureaucratic tool—a means for health system managers to negotiate diverse interests competing for health care resources. By turning to the evidence for what works and what doesn't, managers can make decisions about whose interests to prioritize in specific situations in a politically palatable way—that is, without having to make a substantive ethical commitment to one group's interests versus another's.

> 2-10: 'I think the current central position stems from its role as a currency in negotiating on a society level the interest, the different interests of people in the health care profession or in health care provision.'

Occasionally, participants drew parallels between EBM and religious movements. One participant (3-1) saw EBM as 'objectively wrong', while others believed that trust or faith in EBM was required to be an evidence-based practitioner, as the validity of the evidence hierarchy had never been proven, nor had it ever been shown that evidence-based practice led to improved patient care.

2-6: 'Nobody has ever done a randomized trial . . . this is a great irony of EBM . . . nobody has ever done a randomized trial to randomly assign people to have practitioners in an EBM way and a non-EBM way . . . So I have to take it on faith.'

2.3.5 What is Evidence?

The questions of how to define evidence, and how EBM defines evidence, were of varying degrees of importance to each group. EBM developers largely endorsed the evidence hierarchy as both a valid and a sufficiently broad enumeration of sources of evidence. Some participants expressed the concern that EBM is often misunderstood as only taking RCT data into consideration, when in fact the hierarchy is quite specific that there are many possible sources of evidence to bring to bear upon clinical decisions and that one must use the best available source.

1-3: '. . . it's really providing the best care we can for our patients based on what we know through systematic research rather than just our own anecdotal observations or things that people have told us that we haven't really confirmed to be true about management of patients and, you know, understanding that there are all sorts of sources of evidence. It's not just randomized clinical trials. It's all sorts.'

2.3.6 A False Notion of Evidence

However, many mental health experts and philosophers found that EBM's notion of evidence was too narrow a concept. Some expressed the concern that EBM's concept of evidence was not only narrow but had the potential to convey a false notion of evidence.

2-1: 'There's a notion that, as *The X-Files* would put it, "the truth is out there": a truth to be uncovered, and experimental observation and deduction of hypotheses is the method of uncovering reasoning—that reason is very important and this is the whole enlightenment value that permeates through scientific inquiry to the current day.'

Philosophers viewed evidence as the central concept of EBM and did not view EBM as a tripartite structure that placed clinical expertise and patients' values on an equal footing. In fact, some argued that for EBM to be a substantive concept, it had to prioritize evidence and the evidence hierarchy over other considerations.

3-10: '. . . under that definition I could know all of the medical literature, right? And I go into practice and I base every one of my decisions based on my clinical gut instinct. I know all the literature, right? I just don't weigh it very heavily. I'm integrating it but I'm just, I'm bringing it in with a very low weighting and I'm emphasizing,

I'm weighting heavily my clinical expertise. I could still claim under that definition to be an evidence-based medicine practitioner. But, I'm not sure that anybody else would see you as that and if they would then I'm not sure what the difference is between an evidence-based and a non-evidence-based practitioner.'

3-6: 'I think from the point of view of evidence-based practitioners, if they go too far down all they're asking is for the best available evidence, you start saying: "Well, in what way is that different from what people were saying 20 years earlier?" And those clinicians who got very angry . . . felt the evidence-based medicine people were saying: "You've always practised on the basis of poor evidence and you've been practising lousily and now we're coming along and telling you how you practise." And those people who felt upset by that might reasonably challenge the evidence-based medicine person and say: "Tell us how we haven't been practising on the base of evidence. We've had all sorts of evidence." To which the reply reasonably might have been: "Yeah, but the evidence is not high-quality evidence. It's not an RCT." So in some ways I think if the evidence-based medicine people don't highlight the very high-quality evidence it starts to be no different from, you know, apple pie and motherhood saying: "Well you ought to do whatever seems best on the information you can possibly get." '

At the same time, some group 3 participants found the evidence hierarchy to be a philosophically indefensible concept, as it suggested that there was a correct route to knowledge in all similar situations. To these participants, a correct route to knowledge could not logically be predetermined.

2.3.7 The Practice of EBM Compared to the Five Steps

2.3.7.1 Integration: The Key Step?

In *Evidence-based medicine,* Straus and colleagues begin with the statement that 'Evidence-based medicine requires the integration of the best research evidence with our clinical expertise and our patient's unique values and circumstances' (2011: 1). As mentioned above, these authors believe that doing, using, and replicating modes all count as evidence-based practice because integration occurs in each mode. By what process exactly does the practitioner integrate evidence with clinical expertise and patient values? Some EBM developers believed it involves weighing up the three components of evidence, expertise, and patients' values.

1-2: 'Integration means being able to consider all those three components [evidence, expertise, and patients' values] that I talked about, so not just relying on one aspect, so not just saying, "based on my clinical experience this is what we're going to do"; so it's being able to think about all three of those pieces and sometimes one of those pieces weighs more heavily than the others.'

However, another EBM developer stated that the integration process was unknown and that EBM did not have much to say about it.

1-4: 'Well that's where the mystery begins. We don't know in that decision-making process how to put that together. That's why . . . it's a black box that includes patients' wishes, clinical judgement, the circumstances of the patient, and what we know about the treatments. And evidence-based medicine doesn't have much to say about that. Now the people who are involved in evidence-based medicine are trying to figure that out but I don't think anybody can honestly say they understand all those dimensions and that's where I guess professionalism takes over, whatever that is, the art of medicine and so on. But if you're trying to describe that or trying to look to evidence-based medicine to tell you what's going on I don't think that's conceivable. We don't know how to do that. All we can do is hope that what the medical profession has to offer is a reasonable way, or the best way, we know of to do that.'

In describing integration, none of the interviewees—including EBM developers— mentioned the four questions listed in Figure 2.1, nor did they discuss the quantitative process of clinical decision analysis or LHH described in the texts and reviewed here in Section 2.2.3.3. It seems that the process through which integration takes place remains unsettled. This led one participant to point out that if EBM does not sufficiently define integration, the practitioner will have no way to determine what does and does not count as evidence-based practice.

3-10: 'The patient has ARDS [acute respiratory distress syndrome]. And low-tidal-volume ventilation, we'll all agree, clinical research shows that that's better for outcomes. But every time I put him on low-tidal-volume ventilation he goes into a malignant arrhythmia and he drops his blood pressure and he looks like we're going to have to code him, but if I put him on higher-tidal volume he does okay in terms of his heart. So now my understanding of that circumstance, my pathophysiologic rationale, that malignant arrhythmia is bad for outcome in this individual case, is going to take priority and I'm not going to use the proven therapy of low-tidal-volume ventilation. Is that okay? Does that make me an evidence-based medicine practitioner or not?'

In this example, the participant illustrates the idea that an evidence-based practitioner might be aware of the evidence supporting the use of an intervention, but makes a decision not to use it in light of his clinical judgement based on real-time assessment of the patient. The question this participant raises is how should the practitioner weigh the various considerations, including evidence, in clinical decision-making?

2.3.7.2 Critical Appraisal: The Heart of EBM

Many philosopher/bioethicists saw critical appraisal—step 3—rather than integration, as the heart of EBM. However, they believed that EBM has evolved away from the idea of the individual practitioner engaging in critical appraisal herself towards the use of pre-appraised sources (omitting step 3 from the five steps). While most participants agreed that reliance on pre-appraised evidence sources was good enough evidence-based practice from a clinical point of view, and perhaps even necessary given that critical appraisal was probably too onerous for most clinicians, others viewed the use of pre-appraised sources as an unfortunate compromise that diluted EBM's most powerful, positive, and novel contribution.

> 3-12: '. . . I think that in the early days evidence-based medicine had at its core this idea that people were going to be critically engaged with research. Individual physicians were going to be seeking out the research evidence, they were going to critically analyse it themselves, and they were going to bring that into their practice. And I think that most of that is gone now. I think that the expectation on physicians is that they look up the best available evidence-based guideline on whatever it is that they're worried about and that they follow that.'

> 3-5: '. . . the ethos is not to take these things on trust just because they've been digested for you but actually to do critical appraisal for yourself because after all those things fall out of date even more quickly than the scientific journals and they don't get updated as often as you'd like. And they may not answer the question you need to know the answer to and so it might, for the really purist EBM theorist, be rather like taking your final English literature exam on the basis of the Cliffs Notes.[15] You've got to go back to the sources and check them for yourself. So I think what is good enough and what is really the ideal and the ethos driving evidence-based medicine as a social movement are actually quite far apart.'

2.3.7.3 Evolving

Ultimately, some of the philosophers believed that in its evolution EBM was trying to do too much. A programme that taught clinicians how to find relevant medical research studies (steps 1 and 2) and how to critically appraise them (step 3) seemed to be a philosophically defensible set of ideas. By contrast, integration (step 4) goes beyond evidence and tries to set up an overall model of clinical decision-making, instructing clinicians how to take into account other considerations such as patients' values and clinical expertise. Several philosophers worried that EBM's picture of clinical decision-making was incomplete, emphasizing the content required to make decisions without giving adequate attention to the processes of clinical reasoning in which diagnoses are ruled in or out, or conflicting warrants for action are weighed. Without greater specification, EBM is difficult to define and thus difficult to defend.

----

[15] Cliffs Notes are study guides that in the case of English literature, will summarize a work as well as provide notes, pose questions, and offer tips to understand the primary source.

2.4 **What is EBM? Reprise**

As was clear from the preceding section, even among experts there was a spectrum of views about what actually constitutes EBM. This spectrum ranged from the textbook definition, to a more general idea that emphasizes using research data in clinical care, to the idea that EBM is an unsubstantive term whose content is vague and keeps shifting.

Critics highlighted this lack of clarity and pointed out the conundrum that EBM's authors find themselves in with respect to the definition of EBM. If EBM, as the current definition reads, attempts to integrate a variety of factors in clinical decision-making such as clinical expertise and patients' values without defining integration, couldn't anyone who says that they considered these factors argue that they were engaged in evidence-based practice, regardless of what decision was made? How can this be meaningfully distinguished from the kind of practice that existed prior to the emergence of EBM? In fact, when participants were queried on this point, across all groups they pointed to the application of research data from properly conducted clinical empirical research in accordance with the evidence hierarchy as the important distinguishing feature between pre-EBM and evidence-based practice. Thus, despite protestations, EBM really is about evidence rather than about anything else. Furthermore, according to experts' views, if EBM wants to say something meaningful, it ought to be about evidence and about better-quality evidence (i.e. RCT data) in particular. This point is congruent with the content of EBM textbooks that are largely devoted to ascertaining the quality of research studies. However, others argued that if there is going to be a priority placed on research data, the justification of the evidence hierarchy needed to be developed further.

This focus on the evidence hierarchy hints at why EBM is sometimes understood as being exclusively focused on RCT data. Those commentators who interpret EBM as being RCT-centred may see the evidence hierarchy as the substantial contribution of EBM. Conceiving of EBM as a tripartite structure (evidence, patients' values, and clinical expertise) in which these three inputs are integrated according to some unspecified process may not seem to be novel or different compared to pre-EBM practice. As a result, they focus on what is novel: the prioritization of RCT data by the evidence hierarchy.

2.4.1 **Areas of Uncertainty**

Comparing the textbook definitions of EBM and evidence with experts' definitions has exposed some areas of uncertainty. There are others that were not discussed by the participants but are relevant to understanding how EBM works in practice. For example, the evidence base concerning a given clinical question is constantly in evolution, and for any critical appraisal she does, the clinician will find herself faced with certain questions: how does one handle conflicting data; what quantity of data is enough to support a change to one's clinical practice; and how should one handle data that come from methods not listed on the hierarchy of evidence (such as qualitative studies, intersubjective experience)?

Users' guides mentions the first two issues in passing (Guyatt et al. 2008: 569, 305). On the topic of conflicting data, the authors present possible reasons for conflict such as differences in study participants, interventions, outcomes, and methods. They recommend that practitioners exercise caution in recommending treatments when there is 'large, unexplained heterogeneity' [in the context of meta-analyses]. On the topic of the appropriate amount of data, the authors suggest that clinicians should '. . . wait until a sufficient number of studies showing a sufficient number of events have been conducted before exposing your patients to inconvenient, costly, or potentially risky interventions'. In both cases, the authors indirectly call upon readers to exercise their judgement in determining whether problems in the data are serious and when mitigating circumstances arise.

It is unclear where the exercise of individual judgement belongs in the model of EBM. Recall that EBM refers to clinical expertise (rather than clinical judgement) where clinical expertise is defined as: '. . . the ability to use our clinical skills and past experience to rapidly identify each patient's unique health state and diagnosis, their individual risks and benefits of potential interventions, and their personal values and expectations'. Clinical expertise does not refer to exercising judgement in assessing research data, even though this seems to be what the authors recommend when faced with conflicting or insufficient data. Pre-appraised sources hide judgement even further because the authors of such resources exercise their judgement in ways that are not necessarily transparent to the individual reader. Furthermore, relying on pre-appraised sources, and the judgements of their authors, does seem to lead the clinician back to a kind of dependence on authority that EBM had set out to change.

A final area of uncertainty that will be of particular importance to the ethical analysis of EBM concerns the place of values in the model. EBM sets out to be an approach to clinical decision-making and includes patients' values as part of its practice. However, there is very little mention of other values: those of clinicians, significant others, society, the health system, etc. How do these bear upon evidence-based practice? This question is explored in Chapters 6 and 7. At this point it is worth noting that, with a few exceptions, the texts are largely silent on these issues.

2.5 **Conclusions**

In order to investigate the ethics of EBM and evidence-based psychiatry we need to have some clarity about what these terms mean. The investigation of the meanings of EBM and evidence in this chapter revealed certain important areas of tension. First, is EBM the mastery of research methods and the various computations needed to extrapolate research data? Or is it a process by which these skills are used alongside clinical expertise and patients' values? In the absence of a clear definition of integration, how do we distinguish between evidence-based practice and non-evidence-based practice? Second, is evidence only what is spelled out by the evidence hierarchy? If so, what does this say about kinds of evidence not listed on the hierarchy? Third, if consulting pre-appraised evidence-based resources counts as evidence-based practice, does individual critical appraisal become superfluous? If so, why do the texts devote so much attention to these skills?

These questions have generated extensive, sometimes vitriolic, debate. Chapter 3 reviews and discusses this debate.

References

Evidence-Based Medicine Working Group (1992), 'Evidence-based medicine: a new approach to teaching the practice of medicine', *Journal of the American Medical Association*, **268**: 2420–5.

Ghali, W. A., Saitz, R., Sargious, P. M., and Hershman, W. Y. (1999), 'Evidence-based medicine and the real world: understanding the controversy', *Journal of Evaluation in Clinical Practice*, **5**: 133–8.

Grossman, J., and Mackenzie, F. J. (2005), 'The randomized controlled trial: gold standard or merely standard?' *Perspectives in Biology and Medicine*, **48**: 516–34.

Guyatt, G., Haynes, B., Jaeschke R., Cook, D., Greenhalgh, T., Meade, M., Green, L., Naylor, C. D., Wilson, M., McAlister, F., and Richardson, W. S. (2002), 'The philosophy of evidence-based medicine', in Guyatt, G. and Rennie, D. (eds.), *Users' guides to the medical literature: a manual for evidence-based clinical practice*, 1st edn. (Chicago: AMA Press), 3–12.

Guyatt, G., Rennie, D., Meade, M., and Cook, D. (2008) (eds.), *Users' guides to the medical literature: a manual for evidence-based clinical practice*, 2nd edn. (Chicago: AMA Press).

Haynes, R. B. (2002), 'What kind of evidence is it that evidence-based medicine advocates want health care providers and consumers to pay attention to?' *BMC Health Services Research*, **2** (3): 6 March <http://www.biomedcentral.com/1472-6963/2/3> accessed 27 January 2014.

Hitt, J. (2001), 'The year in ideas: A to Z; evidence-based medicine', *New York Times*, 12 December <http://www.nytimes.com/2001/12/09/magazine/the-year-in-ideas-a-to-z-evidence-based-medicine.html?scp=4&sq=evidence%20based%20medicine&st= cse> accessed 21 April 2009.

Morrison, S. (2007), 'McMaster breakthrough ranks as a top medical milestone', *Daily News*, 9 January <http://dailynews.mcmaster.ca/story.cfm?id=4423> accessed 16 June 2009.

Noseworthy, T. and Watanabe, M. (1999), *'Health policy directions for evidence-based decision-making in Canada'*, *Journal of Evaluation in Clinical Practice*, 5: 227–42.

Straus, S. E., Richardson, W. S., Glasziou, P., and Haynes, R. B. (2005) (eds.), *Evidence-based medicine: how to practice and teach EBM*, 3rd edn. (Edinburgh: Elsevier Churchill Livingstone).

Straus, S. E., Richardson, W. S., Glasziou, P., and Haynes, R. B. (2011) (eds.), *Evidence-based medicine: how to practice and teach EBM*, 4th edn. (Edinburgh: Elsevier Churchill Livingstone).

Upshur, R. E. G. (2003), 'Are all evidence-based practices alike? Problems in the ranking of evidence', *Canadian Medical Association Journal*, 169: 672–3.

Upshur, R. E. G., Buetow, S., Loughlin, M., and Miles, A. (2006), 'Can academic and clinical journals be in financial conflict of interest situations? The case of evidence-based incorporated', *Journal of Evaluation in Clinical Practice*, 12: 405–9.

Chapter 3

Values and evidence-based medicine: the debate

3.1 A Paradigm Shift?

When evidence-based medicine (EBM) was first introduced to the medical literature, its originators declared that it was a paradigm shift compared to what preceded it (Evidence-Based Medicine Working Group 1992: 2420–1). This claim borrows directly from the language of the philosopher of science, Thomas Kuhn. By 'paradigm', Kuhn meant an 'entire framework of concepts, results and procedures' within which science is conducted (Blackburn 1996: 276). A period of 'revolutionary science' leads to the abandonment of the prevailing paradigm, a period of instability where potential new paradigms are in competition, and finally restabilization with the acceptance of a new paradigm. Given this characterization of paradigm, there are those who question whether EBM constitutes a change of this magnitude from its predecessor. First, these authors argue that EBM is not a new development because modern clinical practice has always relied upon scientific evidence of some sort (Benitez-Bribiesca 1999), as opposed to forms of practice that appealed to theory, religion, etc. Second, the fundamental tenets of modern medicine remain unchanged under EBM. In other words, EBM does not challenge the pathophysiological basis of disease; it only challenges pathophysiology as the best basis for evaluating health interventions. In response, EBM advocates argue that the rapid availability of higher-quality research data, in conjunction with the standardization of methods to appraise these data, constitutes a major change from pre-EBM practice. They argue that prior to EBM, evidence included any kind of information (Davidoff et al. 1995; Sackett et al. 1996), and unsubstantiated practice strategies were transmitted and accepted uncritically. More recently, EBM's authors have softened their claim of EBM as a paradigm shift in the Kuhnian sense, but they remain convinced that it is represents a major change to medical practice by emphasizing research data and assigning lower value to clinical experience, pathophysiological rationale, and authority (Guyatt et al. 2008: 10).

Regardless of whether EBM is, or is not, a paradigm shift in Kuhnian terms, it has provoked a response as widespread as its influence. Endorsements, analyses, and critiques have flowed from a variety of disciplines including philosophy, bioethics, sociology, and, of course, the health professions. Chapter 3 focuses on the debates that are most relevant to questions of values—ethical, social, and professional—and evidence-based practice. It highlights the work of authors who point out the role of values in the generation, interpretation, and dissemination of research data. It also examines the arguments of those who have tried to understand the interpretation of evidence in clinical practice, as well as the integration of evidence with clinical expertise and patients' values.

3.2 The Making of Evidence

EBM rests on an important epistemological claim: that it is the best (most accurate, value-free) route to knowledge about which health interventions are effective. In particular, EBM claims to be better than whatever approach was being used before EBM. *Evidence-based medicine*'s authors cite the results of certain high-profile clinical trials that demonstrated that the drugs under investigation, although believed to be effective, actually caused harm. The Cardiac Arrhythmia Suppression Trial (CAST) demonstrated that the anti-arrhythmic drugs encainide and flecainide, in the acute post-myocardial infarction period, contributed to excess arrhythmia-related mortality rather than reducing it (Straus et al. 2011: 69). The Women's Health Initiative Study demonstrated that hormone replacement therapy actually increased the rate of cardiac events among post-menopausal women rather than decreasing it (Straus et al. 2011: 186). These examples became the standard-bearers for EBM, scientifically, clinically, and ethically. If EBM can be used to identify which interventions really work versus which cause harm, then it offers a powerful scientific resource to ensure that practitioners and patients identify the right interventions for a given clinical problem. If clinicians fail to adhere to EBM's principles, they could end up offering interventions that are potentially ineffective or even harmful.

EBM's epistemological claim thus becomes central to an ethical analysis. The idea that ethical practice depends on EBM rests on whether we can trust in the knowledge obtained using the principles of EBM. But how do we know that these principles are correct? Are EBM and the research methods it values most highly really the best route to knowledge about health interventions? In Section 3.3 I examine some of the most important debates that have challenged EBM's claim of being the best route to knowledge about health. The overall theme of these debates concerns the process of knowledge production and the various factors that influence the production of medical research data. Some of the issues raised are as applicable to psychiatry as they are to other branches of medicine, while other issues are of greater or particular concern to psychiatry. I will draw these distinctions where relevant.

3.3 **The Social Context of Knowledge Production**

Several authors argue that rather than freeing us from biases, research data are themselves created and shaped by various social factors, values, and biases. These factors, such as the impact of the source of funding on research and pub-lication bias, influence the kinds of research data that are produced, dissemi-nated, and available to be incorporated into evidence-based practice. Source of funding bias reflects the influence of the funding source on the types of ques-tions researched, how they are researched, and how relevant the resulting data are for clinical practice. Publication bias reflects various aspects of the social process whereby data are selected for dissemination. In a damning statement about the pernicious impact of source of funding bias, publication bias, and conflicts of interest that affect clinical research data, Marcia Angell, former edi-tor of the *New England Journal of Medicine* writes:

> The problems I've discussed are not limited to psychiatry, although they reach their most florid form there. Similar conflicts of interest and biases exist in virtually every field of medicine, particularly those that rely heavily on drugs or devices. It is simply no longer possible to believe much of the clinical research that is published, or to rely on the judgment of trusted physicians or authoritative medical guidelines.
>
> (Angell 2009)

Sections 3.3.1 and 3.3.2 on source of funding bias and publication bias examine how these have the potential to distort clinical research.

3.3.1 **Source of Funding Bias**

Medical research is typically funded in one of three ways: by companies researching products to bring to commercial markets, by philanthropic organizations or foundations, and by governments through nationally funded research councils. Any funder—whether public or private—has priorities and values that inform the types of research and researchers it chooses to fund. In theory, public funders' values are supposed to align with society's values, although the extent to which this occurs or is even possible is unclear. After all, what are society's values and who determines them? Private funders' values will align with the values of those whose money it is. A pharmaceutical company's mandate is to generate profits for its shareholders; therefore, its priorities will be to develop products that will maximize profit. A private foundation will try to fund research that is compatible with the values or vision of the per-son or group who created the foundation. As a result, there will certainly be at least some variance between the kinds of research questions that patients want answered, and the kinds of questions that funders decide are worthy of receiving research funding. In this discussion I will focus on pharmaceutical company funding, as this is the single largest source of funding of clinical trials in psychiatry (Perlis et al. 2005).

3.3.1.1 Business Interests versus Therapeutic Interests

Pharmaceutical companies have the potential to influence the production of evidence in a variety of ways.[1] First, studies of interventions with potential commercial value (e.g. medications or devices) will be funded by the businesses that stand to profit, unlike those interventions that have no such commercial value. The latter group includes both interventions that will not yield great profits and interventions that might be quite effective but do not have a sufficiently large market; this is the case for rare conditions or conditions that primarily affect people without the financial means to pay for the intervention. As a result, there tends to be a much larger body of evidence about commercially valuable interventions.

Second, the majority of clinical trials are designed to meet funders' business interests—that is, to achieve regulatory approval and market access (Healy 2001). This means that industry-funded trials will be designed to maximize the chances that the trial will successfully fulfil the requirements of regulators—namely, that new products have a greater effect on outcome than placebo. On the other hand, clinicians and patients may have very different questions that need answering. Faced with having to make a treatment recommendation, a clinician may want to know whether a product is better than other available treatments rather than whether it is better than placebo. A patient may want to know what the effect of a drug is on a person like himself, rather than like the participants typically recruited to clinical trials. For example, patients enrolled in randomized controlled trials (RCTs) in psychiatry usually have one disorder (e.g. depression), unlike patients in real practice who commonly have several, potentially overlapping disorders or symptoms (e.g. depression, anxiety, substance abuse). Follow-up in RCTs of pharmaceutical agents is often short-term (weeks), while the actual duration and treatment of mental disorders is usually long-term (years). Choosing certain parameters, such as short-term follow-up

---

[1] There is a rich body of literature that has explored the impact of industry funding on clinical trial results, including in psychiatry. See, for example, Bhandari et al. 2004; Kelly Jr. et al. 2006; Schott et al. 2010, and Sismondo 2008. My aim in this section is not to try to validate these claims. Instead, I wish to point out the mechanisms by which funders can influence trials and trial data, and the values that underlie their actions.

and less complex patients, makes it simpler for companies to demonstrate that an experimental drug does or does not have an effect greater than placebo. However, given the complex, comorbid, and chronic nature of mental disorder, it is unclear what these short-term, internally valid[2] RCTs can contribute to clinical decision-making involving specific individuals.

Third, techniques used by commercial funders such as ghost-writing[3] and detailing[4] further accelerate and amplify the influence of industry-sponsored research data compared with non-industry-funded data within the evidence base. EBM is about using the medical literature to determine which interventions are supported by the best evidence, but source of funding bias creates the potential for the medical literature to be heavily skewed towards RCT data used for the regulatory approval of commercially valuable interventions over non-commercially valuable data (De Vries and Lemmens 2006: 2696–7).

3.3.1.2 *Users' Guides* and Source of Funding Bias

The current edition of *Users' guides* (Guyatt et al. 2008) includes a chapter entitled 'Dealing with misleading presentations of clinical trial results'. This focuses on the second issue discussed in the previous section—that for-profit funders seek to advance their business interests by setting up trials and analysing and presenting trial data in certain ways. The *Users' guides* chapter goes on to offer eight guides to help the reader avoid being misled by these practices (Guyatt et al. 2008: 303).

It is certainly worthwhile for the authors of *Users' guides* to note that the presentation of research data contains a persuasive element in which the reader is led to draw certain conclusions. Further, it is important that the authors point out that the motive of for-profit funders in presenting data in certain ways is to encourage readers to prescribe their products. However, there are two major omissions in this approach that reflect the authors' underlying belief about the

---

[2] Internal validity refers to the extent to which a research study has accurately discerned the true direction and magnitude of the effect of the intervention under investigation, and is affected by many aspects of study design. Testing new treatments in groups with single psychiatric diagnoses, as is common practice in clinical trials, allows researchers to draw conclusions about the effect of the intervention on that disorder without having to worry about the influence of other symptoms or disorders.

[3] Ghost-writing is the practice by which industry-sponsored trials are reported in academic publications that list academic physicians as the principal authors when in fact the papers are written by industry-paid writers.

[4] Detailing is the practice whereby pharmaceutical sales representatives visit prescribers to discuss company products.

value-neutrality of EBM. First, by focusing only on the presentation of data, the authors fail to locate this issue within the larger context of the social process of knowledge production. In other words, the problem is not only that data may be presented in certain ways but also that certain kinds of research questions are never asked and certain kinds of data are never produced. Readers ought to be equally aware of these issues and how they shape what is published in the medical literature. A second omission is that framing the problem as one of identifying and seeing through 'misleading' presentations of data fails to acknowledge that all presentations of data are designed to invite certain conclusions. In other words, all data are presented in ways that suit the interests, values, and aims of the presenter. And all interpretations are made through the lens of the interests, values, and aims of the interpreter, including the critical appraiser who is adhering to the rules of EBM. This does not mean that all interpretations are equally sound, merely that there is no stance that can underwrite a neutral interpretation.

3.3.1.3 Source of Funding Bias in Psychiatry

Source of funding bias is as important in psychiatry as it is in other areas of medicine in terms of potentially facilitating the widespread dissemination of misleading information about interventions with commercial value. However, there are reasons why psychiatrists should be particularly concerned about it. Angell (2011) has argued that psychiatry is particularly vulnerable to the types of distortions in published research data that can arise through industry funding of research. Because the pathophysiology of mental disorders is unknown and not verifiable using the standard objective methods of the rest of medicine (physical exam, lab results, imaging), industry sponsors are more able to extend, manipulate, or even create diagnostic categories in order to create market niches for their products in a way they are less able to in other specialties. A manufacturer can extend a psychiatric diagnostic category, test a product on people who fit into this extended category, and, if successful, claim that its product treats this newly-defined problem. Who is to say otherwise? In other areas of medicine, such an approach is more difficult because there are often accepted physical definitions of what constitutes abnormality.[5] Angell points out that the success of these industry influences has been propelled by a receptive audience of psychiatrists. The profession has its own interests: ideological (a desire to appear as much like the rest of medicine as

---

[5] Although even other areas of medicine can be vulnerable to diagnostic manipulation, such as the transformation of risk factors into disease states that require treatment (Moynihan et al. 2002).

possible) and competitive (with other mental health care providers). These interests have compromised its ability to remain impartial about the effectiveness of psychiatric interventions. The confluence of professional interests and industry influence, particularly as it concerns the uptake of new psychiatric medications, remains an area of enormous ethical concern, and the role of EBM in this process is not benign. By encouraging practitioners to rely heavily on medical research studies to guide their practice, while simultaneously paying relatively little attention to source of funding bias and the economic conditions that foster it, EBM is implicated in the way that its calls for the best evidence can lead to a systematically distorted view of mental disorders and their treatments.

3.3.2 Publication Bias

Publication bias refers to the preferential publication in medical journals of positive and/or statistically significant results rather than negative ones (Gilbody and Song 2000).[6] As a result, the total body of data that could be considered as evidence is narrowed because only certain data are disseminated to practitioners through the medical literature. For example, in a recent paper Turner and colleagues (2008) determined that the majority of negative trials concerning several antidepressants had never been published. Publication bias may result from various decisions along the entire chain of knowledge production. First, publication bias can lead researchers to neglect entire topics: because publications count significantly towards their career advancement (Miettinen 1998), researchers may choose to study the restricted group of topics most likely to yield positive results. Second, researchers may believe their chances of publishing their data are higher if they report only the positive outcomes or if they abandon studies that yield only negative results. Third, as Lexchin and colleagues (2003) have argued, data generated by commercial funders are more likely to demonstrate the effectiveness of the sponsored intervention than data generated by non-commercial funders. Therefore, what is submitted for publication may already be influenced by factors such as which outcome measures are reported, what agents are chosen as comparators, and at what doses. In addition, private companies may choose not to submit data for publication that they do not wish to see enter the public domain, such as data showing negative results or harm. Through publication bias clinicians may thus be exposed to studies that misleadingly suggest the superiority of

---

[6] Positive results show that there is a statistically significant difference in the effect of the study intervention compared to the control intervention. Negative results show that there is no such difference.

certain interventions. Finally, journals have an interest in selling subscriptions and reprints (Spielmans and Parry 2010), and may wish to make their content more interesting to practitioners by publishing studies where the interventions under investigation are shown to be effective.

3.3.2.1 Detecting Publication Bias

EBM's authors have been more attentive to publication bias than source of funding bias. For example, *Users' guides* devotes a chapter to publication bias (or 'reporting bias' as it is called in the book), particularly as it manifests in systematic reviews and meta-analyses (Guyatt et al. 2008: 543–54). The authors emphasize various techniques and tests that the EBM practitioner can use to detect publication bias, although they acknowledge that these are useful only in a minority of situations. The *Users' guides* chapter concludes with a call for comprehensive clinical trial registries[7] that would, at the very least, make it more difficult to avoid publishing negative clinical trial data. However, the chapter gives little consideration to the web of social and economic interests—journal, researcher, and funder—that makes positive results so important. The *Users' guide* authors take the position that technical solutions and rules can mitigate these interests rather than addressing the reasons they exist in the first place.

Others have also pointed to a clinical trial registry as a possible solution to the problem of publication bias (Moher 1993; Chalmers et al. 1992). A register of all clinical trials intended or underway could ensure that it would not be possible to hold back trial data from the public domain. Under this scheme, when preparing systematic reviews authors would demonstrate that they examined data emerging from all relevant registered trials, rather than merely those that were published. To date several national, international, and corporate registers exist. In addition, the International Committee of Medical Journal Editors (ICMJE) has introduced clinical trial registration as part of their uniform requirements for manuscripts in member journals. However, the extent to which these developments will decrease the impact of publication bias remains to be seen. Mathieu and colleagues (2009) found that in spite of the introduction of this requirement in 2005, by 2008 inadequate registration (registration after the trial and/or without specification of the primary

---

[7] A registry is a database of ongoing clinical trials. Registries can contain quite detailed information about the trial, including the entire protocol. See, for example, <http://www.ClinicalTrials.gov> (accessed 29 January 2014), which is an American government-sponsored registry of publicly and privately supported clinical trials of new drugs.

outcome) and discrepancies between the registered primary outcome and the published data were still common.

3.4 Values in the Hierarchy of Evidence

The debate about source of funding bias and publication bias has identified ways in which the process of knowledge production can lead to distortions in the generation of evidence. This debate calls into question whether the evidence held up by EBM really can be relied upon to tell us what works. Proponents of EBM might acknowledge that these biases are indeed a problem, but they argue that they are external to EBM and are not the fault of EBM per se. According to this argument, these biases are merely contingent factors and the basic principles and concepts of EBM, including the evidence hierarchy, are truth-orientated.

Nevertheless, some scholars have expressed concerns about the various ways in which EBM's own methods can go wrong. For example, they highlight methodological and statistical problems that plague RCTs and meta-analyses of RCTs (Eysenck 1991; Feinstein and Horwitz 1997; Grossman and McKenzie 2005; Horwitz 1996; Lau et al. 1998). According to these authors, poor study design and faulty execution yield flawed data that cannot be considered valid and from which accurate inferences cannot be drawn. Proponents of EBM acknowledge that poor-quality research limits validity of data and have called for better-designed studies (Miké 1999) but stick to the idea that EBM's rules are not flawed; rather, some researchers design flawed studies. If researchers improved their study designs, RCTs would deserve their place at the top of the hierarchy.

EBM's authors remind us that the hierarchy of evidence is the first 'fundamental principle' of EBM (Guyatt et al. 2008: 10). It is the hierarchy that directs clinicians' attention towards certain kinds of research while encouraging them to dismiss others. And the hierarchy is the basis of EBM's claim that it is the best route to securing knowledge about what really works by prioritizing randomized controlled double-blind trials (or systematic reviews of such trials) while designating other research methods as inferior. In the absence of a hierarchy, we are back to a situation in which medical research studies of various types are disseminated to clinical audiences without a clear set of directions about which ones are the most important. Without the hierarchy, EBM does not seem to be distinct from what existed before EBM. Sections 3.4.1 and 3.4.2 discuss arguments that question this basic principle of EBM, including the placement of the RCT at the top of the evidence hierarchy. Like the debates about knowledge production, these arguments challenge EBM's claim of being the best route to knowledge.

3.4.1 Is Randomization Necessary?

Randomization is the process by which study participants are assigned to either a treatment or a control group purely on the basis of chance. Randomization allegedly balances both known and unknown confounding variables,[8] both eliminating the need for researchers to judge which known confounders ought to be balanced and eliminating worries about unknown confounders (Worrall 2010). By eliminating the impact of confounding variables, randomization is advocated by EBM proponents as essential to ensure that trials isolate the impact of the intervention under investigation. However, there has been important debate on this point (Urbach 1993; Worrall 2002; 2004; 2010). Worrall (2004) argues that randomization will only lead to balanced groups (in which one group does not systematically including a confounding variable) with infinite replications of a trial, and that in any one experiment there will probably be confounding variables that are distributed in an unbalanced way between groups on the basis of chance. Furthermore, since some confounders are acknowledged to be unknown, there is no way of knowing whether this has happened in any specific trial. The main value of randomization is that it can eliminate selection bias—not through the randomization process itself, but because the allocation to study groups is concealed in a randomized design. He points out that the same goal can be achieved through blinding (Worrall 2010). Worrall makes a connection between the insistence on the necessity of randomization and ethics. He points out that because of randomization patients assigned to control groups may be exposed to hazards in the name of methodological superiority, even when lower-ranked methods can be relied upon to show that the control condition is therapeutically inferior (2002).[9]

Along with Worrall, several scholars have challenged the notion of the primacy of the RCT and, therefore, the hierarchy of evidence itself. Bluhm (2009) has questioned the automatic privileging of RCTs over other study designs, arguing that non-randomized studies can achieve the goals of balance in confounding variables between treatment and control groups. She also argues that

---

[8] A confounding variable or confounder is one that is associated with the outcome but is systematically differentially distributed between study groups.

[9] Worrall explores a specific case from the 1980s of extracorporeal membraneous oxygenation (ECMO) for neonates suffering from persistent pulmonary hypertension. He argues that in spite of evidence from historical controls and a clinical trial with a modified randomization protocol, researchers conducted a prospective RCT out of a belief that this was necessary to provide convincing evidence of treatment superiority. During the course of the trial four control group babies receiving conventional therapy died.

observational-type designs may be more useful in many cases because of practical advantages such as longer duration of follow-up (in other words, observational designs have greater external validity[10]). In response, Howick (2011) has argued that a randomized design need only be able to rule out more confounders than other types of studies to deserve its place at the top of the hierarchy. Further, he notes that if a study lacks internal validity because of bias it cannot be saved by a high degree of external validity. However, Borgerson (2009) has pointed out that there are many types of bias, not only the ones that are directly addressed by randomization and double-blinding. She argues that the RCT design does not uniquely remove all relevant biases; thus, RCTs do not have a special claim to causal knowledge. Indeed, RCTs themselves are prone to particular biases that will be discussed in more detail in the next section.

3.4.2 Technical Bias of the Evidence Hierarchy

Technical bias reflects our tendency to measure what we are able to measure, thus privileging research data that we know how to obtain and/or can obtain easily. As a result, any method or approach can offer only a partial view of what it is trying to study, as certain aspects of a phenomenon will be captured by that method and not others. Culpepper and Gilbert (1999) point out that the evidence hierarchy privileges certain types of research methodologies and, therefore, the data (evidence) that these methodologies produce. By contrast, phenomena not easily amenable to investigation by the privileged methods may be neglected or presumed unworthy of inquiry compared to those interventions best suited to the preferred methods (Kerridge et al. 1998: 1151–2). For example, 'practical evidence' (interpretation of experience) and clinical information derived from intuition and judgement in the clinical encounter are examples of knowledge that have, to date, been poorly integrated into EBM's evidence (Buetow and Kenealy 2000; Knottnerus and Dinant 1997; Malterud 1995; Tanenbaum 1993). These phenomena could perhaps be better understood through a variety of research strategies, including qualitative methods that are given only peripheral consideration by EBM proponents.[11] By requiring

---

[10] External validity refers to the extent to which research results can be generalized to a population or setting other than the one that was studied.

[11] Numerous scholars have suggested the inclusion of other research methods into the evidence hierarchy, whether qualitative (Barbour 2000; Dixon-Woods et al. 2001; Green and Britten 1998; Upshur 2001) or conceptual (Berkwits 1998). *Users' guides* does contain a chapter on critically appraising qualitative research, while *Evidence-based medicine* contains a section (Guyatt et al. 2008; Straus et al. 2011). Although these inclusions suggest the authors' openness to these concerns, qualitative research receives fairly minimal coverage relative to the length of both works.

every medical phenomenon in the domains of diagnosis, prognosis, treatment, and harm to be investigated using EBM-preferred research methods, it is quite likely that some of these phenomena are not being very well investigated at all. The possibility that one might have to use non-EBM-preferred methods to generate data of *better* quality is never considered.

Alternatively, some phenomena may be subject to investigation by EBM, yet the methods of EBM are inadequate to investigate them properly (Kerridge et al. 1998). Psychodynamic psychotherapy, a mainstay of psychiatric practice for decades, has suffered in the EBM era because of the difficulties in devising studies that would meet the methodological demands of EBM-preferred research methods such as RCTs. Where phenomena are a poor fit for EBM-preferred methods, the interventions under investigation seem doomed to be inadequately evidence-based in perpetuity. For example, an RCT of psychodynamic psychotherapy would have to distort the intervention so much in order to adhere to the methodological demands of EBM that it may no longer be a study of what practitioners actually do when they practise this type of therapy. If, on the other hand, this type of therapy could be studied using some alternate research design less favoured by EBM, according to the logic of the evidence hierarchy, the evidence in support of this intervention would always be considered tentative because an RCT had not been performed. Psychodynamic psychotherapy may, or may not, be an effective form of practice in various clinical situations, but EBM will make it difficult to draw a conclusion either way, leaving it in perpetual limbo. Compared to treatments that are easier to research using the EBM approach, it is plausible that treatments that are more difficult to research will gradually become marginalized in clinical practice. Technical bias has the potential to skew the total pool of evidence in favour of interventions that are easy to investigate using EBM-preferred methods and thus attract more attention, funding, and value in planning clinical services. Likewise, technical bias can skew the evidence base away from interventions or practices that do not easily fit into the EBM conception of research and evidence.

EBM proponents have acknowledged that, by the rules of EBM itself, there is no evidence that EBM is a more effective means of pursuing health than medicine as usual (Norman 1999; Haynes 2002; Straus and McAlister 2000: 839). They point out that it might be difficult to support this claim using EBM-preferred strategies. For example, after more than 20 years of EBM, it would now be difficult to conduct a trial in which the pure intervention (EBM) was offered by the experimental group, but not at all by the control group. In other words, technical bias is so powerful that it prevents EBM from justifying itself. The point here is not to dismiss the hierarchy of evidence because it is biased. Rather, it is to point out that the hierarchy reflects certain scientific values (such as internal validity) that also reflect ethical choices about what kind of knowledge is important and/or necessary when it comes to health. Any approach to knowledge about health will have to make such choices. In claiming to be value-free, EBM does not acknowledge them.

3.5 **From Data to Evidence: The Role of Interpretation**

Recall that EBM rests on an important epistemological claim: adhering to its methods is the best way of having knowledge about which health interventions actually work. Thus far we have examined issues relating to potential biases, distortions, and values in the generation and dissemination of research data. This section examines a different theme: by what process do data become evidence?

A significant body of literature highlights the idea that EBM's epistemological claim obscures the interpretative, and thus subjective, aspect of knowledge generation. EBM's very definition of evidence suggests that data alone will tell us which interventions are, or are not, effective. The definitions of evidence equate it with clinically relevant research (Straus et al. 2011: 1) or any empirical observation (Guyatt et al. 2008: 10). Is evidence the same thing as research or an observation? Consider this claim: 'the perfect synopsis would provide only, and exactly, enough information to support a clinical action' (Straus et al. 2011: 38). But data do not support clinical actions by themselves: someone must first make an interpretation that they do support a clinical action. *Users' guides* does mention interpretation in saying that, in contrast to pre-EBM medicine, EBM 'suggests that interpreting the results of clinical research requires a formal set of rules...' (Guyatt et al. 2008: 10). However, this comment seems to miss the subjective component of interpretation. Interpretation can be structured by rules, but rules cannot fully describe how to interpret: if they did, the result would no longer—by definition—be an interpretation. EBM's jump from observation to data and then to evidence (using rules) seems to ignore the subjective aspect of the process through which data become evidence in support of particular hypotheses.

Goodman asks: 'how should one make an empirical decision under uncertainty when an error might harm someone?' (2005: 552). He argues that it is unethical not to be aware of—and practise according to—evidence-based practice guidelines. However, he recognizes that individual variation exists: that sometimes the practitioner may judge that guidelines are not applicable to a specific patient. In these cases it is incumbent on the practitioner to make the case that deviation from guidelines is necessary. Shahar (1997) points out that it is not merely in cases of potential deviation that doctors ought to be engaging in this type of interpretative judgement. He poses the same question as Goodman: 'one may ask how doctors are to make medical decisions in the presence of permanent uncertainty. The answer is simple: on the basis of some interpretation of empirical experience—a subjective exercise with no universally accepted logical rules' (Shahar 1997: 115).

Downie et al. (2000) argue that in order for something (e.g. data) to be construed as evidence, it must be judged relevant and weighty with respect to some conclusion. It is through this process that data are determined to support certain conclusions. In other words, evidence does not exist on its own; it must be evidence for something, such as a hypothesis or theory. Judgements of whether some datum constitutes 'evidence for' something require interpretation, which may differ between individuals for legitimate reasons (Oakley-Browne 2001; Upshur 1999). Tonelli (2012) points out that study design (the main focus of EBM) is only one of several factors that affect the 'compellingness' of research data. He argues that compellingness arises from as many as 12 different features of clinical research that he groups under three headings: epistemic factors, considerations of individual patient benefit, and attention to stewardship of health care resources.[12] For a given clinician, some or all of these 12 factors will play roles of differing weight when considering whether the data from a particular study could be interpreted as clinically effective. Different assessments of compellingness can lead to different conclusions and variability in practice.

Contrary to EBM's notion of unbiased evidence (evidence that deviates from the truth as little as possible), Upshur states that evidence itself does not constitute truth; rather, evidence plays a role in determining what is believed to be true (personal communication 2001). He points to the legal notion of evidence as a comparison. In a court case, evidence is used to support various theories of what actually happened during a crime. One of these theories is 'discovered', on the basis of the available evidence, to be true. The selection of evidence to support conclusions is negotiated and debated, and is affected by social forces such

---

[12] Tonelli's 12 factors were derived from his participation in a committee of intensive care specialists whose task was to identify the factors through which clinical research reports affect clinical decision-making. They included epistemic (prior knowledge/belief, biological plausibility, consistency/confirmation [relative to other studies on the same topic], objectivity); individual benefit (applicability, effect size, value of outcome, safety, time to effect, alternatives—in relation to comparative effectiveness); and stewardship (cost, ease of implementation, alternatives—in relation to cost) factors.

as the power, coercion, and self-interest of one negotiator or group of negotiators vis-à-vis another. The selection of evidence is also affected by psychological forces, such as faith or psychic comfort, with certain interpretations. These forces may have an impact on which conclusions or theories are ultimately selected to be true.

The recent debate about the effectiveness of antidepressants illustrates the role that compellingness and social and psychological factors play in the transition from data to evidence to practice. This debate also highlights the ethical significance of interpretation. In a controversial 2008 paper, Kirsch and colleagues argued that, taking into account the published and unpublished trial data concerning four antidepressant medications, these drugs showed no benefit over placebo for less depressed patients and only a minor benefit over placebo among severely depressed patients, which was attributable to decreased placebo responsiveness rather than drug effectiveness. Nevertheless, within mainstream psychiatric practice these medications[13] are accepted to be effective in the treatment of major depressive disorder (Lam et al. 2009: S28). Meanwhile, Moncrieff has argued for another possible interpretation: she suggests that a combination of placebo effect and a general drug-induced state produced by the medications accounts for whatever positive effect is noted in these trials rather than any specific pharmacodynamic characteristic attributable to the drugs (2009: 159–73).

This leaves us with three possible interpretations of the impact of these medications: 1) they are effective owing to the active drug ingredient having some specific pharmacodynamic action; 2) they are effective through the placebo effect; and 3) they have a specific mechanism of action that induces a non-specific altered mental state along with a placebo effect. All three interpretations are plausible, but none is self-evidently true or false. It is up to the psychiatric professional community to determine which of these is most likely and, furthermore, which to present to patients seeking treatment for major depression. What will affect theory choice?

The scientific quality of the research—as indicated by study design—will be one factor that influences choice of, and belief in, a theory. EBM's critical

---

[13] These guidelines list three (fluoxetine, venlafaxine and paroxetine) of the medications studied by Kirsch et al. as first-line treatments, meaning they offer the best balance of efficacy, tolerability, and clinical support. Nefazodone was also included in Kirsch and colleagues' (2008) paper, but is not listed by the Canadian Network for Mood and Anxiety Treatments (CANMAT) as it was removed from the Canadian market in 2004.

appraisal rules are relevant to this component of interpretation. However, scientific criteria alone do not settle the dispute. Angell (2011) suggests that both professional and financial interests can, and have, influenced psychiatrists in favour of theory one—specific antidepressant effectiveness. The notion of a professional interest may contain certain aspirations, including a desire to distinguish psychiatry from other mental health care professions, as well as a psychological wish that psychiatric treatments do work and that psychiatrists are really helping their patients. Tonelli's analysis of compellingness is also helpful. Some practitioners might find one interpretation more compelling because it is more consistent with the overall body of knowledge, or more biologically plausible, or easier to implement in actual practice. Ultimately, interpretative choice is ethically significant because it reflects the chooser's attitude towards what kinds of information patients ought to have in making decisions to take medications recommended by psychiatrists.

Considering something to be evidence reflects a subjective judgement that a fact is a warrant to believe a given conclusion in a given situation. For any phenomena, such as the putative effect of antidepressants on depressed people, there may be many available facts that could count as evidence for a conclusion. However, only some facts will be deemed evidence for that conclusion, which itself will be chosen from among several possible conclusions that could be drawn. Thus, evidence is not, as EBM implies, simply research data or facts applied to a scenario, but a series of interpretations that serve and take into account a variety of social, scientific, and ethical factors.

3.6 Integration—EBM in Action

Having looked at some of the issues involved in generating, interpreting, and disseminating research data, which are primarily aspects of the first three steps of evidence-based practice (see Section 2.2), we have arrived at step 4—integration. Integration is the key to EBM, as all three of its modes—doing, using, and replicating—require the practitioner to integrate evidence with clinical expertise and patients' values. EBM texts describe integration as a quantitative process that unfolds through such methods as decision analysis. In essence, integration is the process by which research data are presented to patients whose preferences are quantified and then matched to the probabilities of achieving certain outcomes (both benefits and harms) through the use of available interventions.

Several authors have pointed out that results from large-scale trials cannot be directly applied in situations involving individual patients (Norman 1999: 141; Tonelli 1998: 1238). *Evidence-based medicine* advises readers that whether research data apply to any given patient can be estimated by how similar one's patient is to the trial participants. If dissimilar, one is to judge whether the differences would affect the intervention's effectiveness (Straus et al. 2011: 88–9). These judgements require pathophysiological reasoning; this form of evidence does not even qualify for ranking on the evidence hierarchy, but in this context it is encouraged. *Users' guides* acknowledges that, even if the overall study results show that an intervention is beneficial, some patients will benefit while others may not (just as it is very likely that some study participants benefited while others did not); thus, it may not be possible to judge whether one's actual patient will benefit or not (Guyatt et al. 2008: 180). Both *Evidence-based medicine* and *Users' guides* respond to the problem of application to individual patients by suggesting n-of-1 randomized trials as a solution, but *Users' guides* notes that these can only be conducted under very specific conditions and pose 'considerable logistical challenges' (Guyatt et al. 2008: 11).

Upshur and Colak (2003) argue that the search for research data and their use in justifying clinical recommendations is only one process relevant to clinical practice because clinical encounters are not all of the same type. When interacting with patients who may be seeking information or advice, trying to make decisions, or some combination of these, warrants for action may not be data-based but may be normative or opinion-based, and these warrants may be entirely appropriate for the type of encounter at hand. Different evidentiary standards are required in different circumstances, and the interplay between clinical expertise, values (and/or preferences), and research data is contextually determined. Thus, there may not be a single formula for how to integrate.

In a similar vein, Tonelli (2006) develops the concept of integration by advancing a casuistic model that would lead to the consideration of all types of warrants: 1) empirical evidence; 2) experiential evidence; 3) pathophysiologic rationale; 4) patient goals and values; and 5) system features. He argues that no one type of warrant can automatically be given priority over the others in all cases, and that warrants must be reasoned about and weighed. For Tonelli, integration—conceived of in this way rather than the narrower version offered by EBM—is exactly the skill of medical practice and it includes the capacity to engage in this process explicitly, rigorously, and knowledgeably.

In a later paper he argues that in clinical practice clinicians must be aware of a variety of facts (including research data), but must then use these to argue for or against particular clinical decisions based on whether there is a warrant to apply those facts to the given claim or situation, a warrant being a more general hypothesis that the facts apply in a given case. He points out that 'clinical medicine is a casuistic (case-based) enterprise, personal and prudential, requiring clinicians to weigh and negotiate between multiple potential facts, values, and reasons in order to arrive at the best choice for a particular individual in need of healing' (Tonelli 2009: 322). Tonelli highlights the role that the clinician—via his or her capacity to consider, weigh, and debate; and his or her own values about what is important—necessarily plays in mediating between data and the patient. There can be no direct, rule-driven, or value-neutral path from data to decision. Although EBM outlines a general structure for integration, the details of the process remain unclear and, as the preceding discussion illustrates, this may be because the process is dependent on a variety of individual and contextual factors whose specific manner of being considered in a clinical scenario cannot be determined in advance.

3.7 Conclusions

The preceding discussion does not aim to provide exhaustive coverage of all aspects of the scholarly debate about EBM. However, it does strive to cover the literature concerning the most contentious issues that have arisen in response to the practice of EBM, particularly its self-description as a comprehensive guide to clinical decision-making through its five steps.

Although EBM claims to be a value-neutral approach to practice, the debates discussed here illustrate that every phase of knowledge production, as well as the five steps, is imbued with values, including ethical values. Is EBM's epistemological claim correct? Is it the best way to find out which interventions really work? Or does it actually reflect the ethical values of funders, researchers, and clinicians about what interventions they think are worthwhile, for whom, and in which circumstances? Several questions emerge. What is to be done about the external values that influence knowledge production (source of funding bias, publication bias), and how should practitioners understand and represent the resulting evidence given the impact of these biases? How do the values of the evidence hierarchy affect EBM-type knowledge in daily practice? How should practitioners consider these values and factor them into their conversations with patients and their clinical decisions? If interpretation of research data is irreducibly variable, how should practitioners guard against undue exercise of ethical values in interpretation? Given the many sources of values that are present in generating and disseminating evidence, how can these be meaningfully integrated with patients' values? In examining the debate about EBM, we find that some of the most pressing issues for the clinician trying to practise evidence-based medicine are ethical ones.

The critical debate about EBM has taken an interesting trajectory. When a new criticism emerges, EBM proponents claim the criticism is really a misperception (Straus and McAlister 2000). For example, in EBM's early years, critics accused it of being a cookbook approach that failed to consider individual patient values. In the second edition of *Evidence-based medicine* its authors stated that practising EBM included integrating evidence with patients' values (Sackett et al. 2000: 7–8), even though in the original version they had claimed that practising EBM involved integrating evidence only with clinical expertise (Sackett et al. 1998: 2). Sehon and Stanley (2003) suggest that EBM proponents tend to define EBM as including all that counts as good medical practice, allowing them an inclusive, but empty, response to the question of what exactly EBM is. On the other hand, the sizeable and varied critical responses to EBM suggest that it is not merely a vacuous concept but includes substantive elements—whether stated or implied—regarding the nature of evidence, the process of interpretation, and the process of clinical decision-making.

By claiming a privileged position as an approach to clinical practice based on science, EBM has attracted both adherents and detractors. Its wholesale uptake by the health disciplines reflects the remarkable effectiveness of its spokespeople. However, EBM has also been viciously attacked, including from within the ranks of medicine (Polychronis et al. 1996; Charlton and Miles 1998). Some authors have argued that EBM disguises its intentions as a bid for power by health researchers and academic physicians over frontline practitioners, patients, and research participants (Denny 1999; Ray 1999; Traynor 1999).

The discipline of psychiatry has, in the last generation, been particularly sensitive to questions of its use and abuse of power. Interestingly, it is within psychiatry that the hopes for EBM have been highest: by drawing upon hard scientific data to support their interventions, psychiatrists hope to quell the persistent perception of psychiatric interventions as unscientific and unethical. It is to the field of psychiatry that the next chapter turns.

References

Angell, M. (2009), 'Drug companies and doctors: a story of corruption', *The New York Review of Books*, **56** (1): 15 January <http://www.nybooks.com/articles/22237> accessed 14 December 2013.

Angell, M. (2011), 'The epidemic of mental illness: why?', *The New York Review of Books*, **58** (11): 23 June <http://www.nybooks.com/articles/archives/2011/jun/23/epidemic-mental-illness-why/?pagination=false> accessed 1 January 2013.

Barbour, R. S. (2000), 'The role of qualitative research in broadening the "evidence base" for clinical practice', *Journal of Evaluation in Clinical Practice*, **6**: 155–63.

Benitez-Bribiesca, L. (1999), 'Evidence-based medicine: a new paradigm?' *Archives of Medical Research*, **30**: 77–9.

Berkwits, M. (1998), 'From practice to research: the case for criticism in an age of evidence', *Social Science and Medicine*, **47**: 1539–45.

Bhandari, M., Busse, J. W., Jackowski, D., Montori, V. M., Schünemann, H., Sprague, S., Mears, D., Schemitsch, E. H., Heels-Ansdell, D., and Devereaux P. J. (2004), 'Association between industry funding and statistically significant pro-industry findings in medical and surgical randomized trials', *Canadian Medical Association Journal*, **170**: 477–80.

Blackburn, S. (1996), *Oxford dictionary of philosophy* (Oxford: Oxford University Press).

Bluhm, R. (2009), 'Some observations on "observational" research', *Perspectives in Biology and Medicine*, **52**: 252–63.

Borgerson, K. (2009), 'Valuing evidence: bias and the evidence hierarchy of evidence-based medicine', *Perspectives in Biology and Medicine*, **52**: 218–33.

Buetow, S. and Kenealy, T. (2000), 'Evidence-based medicine: the need for a new definition', *Journal of Evaluation in Clinical Practice*, **6**: 85–92.

Chalmers, I., Dickersin, K., and Chalmers, T. (1992), 'Getting to grips with Archie Cochrane's agenda: all randomized controlled trials should be registered and reported', *British Medical Journal*, **305**: 786–7.

Charlton, B. G. and Miles, A. (1998), 'The rise and fall of EBM', *Quarterly Journal of Medicine*, **91**: 371–4.

Culpepper, L. and Gilbert, T. T. (1999), 'Evidence and ethics', *The Lancet*, **353**: 829–31.

Davidoff, F., Case, K., and Fried, P. W. (1995), 'Evidence-based medicine: why all the fuss?' *Annals of Internal Medicine*, **122**: 727.

Denny, K. (1999), 'Evidence-based medicine and authority', *Journal of Medical Humanities*, **20**: 247–63.

De Vries, R. and Lemmens, T. (2006), 'The social and cultural shaping of medical evidence: case studies from pharmaceutical research and obstetric science', *Social Science & Medicine*, **62**: 2694–706.

Dixon-Woods, M., Fitzpatrick, R., and Roberts, K. (2001), 'Including qualitative research in systematic reviews: opportunities and problems', *Journal of Evaluation in Clinical Practice*, **7**: 125–33.

Downie, R. S. and MacNaughton, J. with Randall, F. (2000), 'Judgment and science', in: *Clinical judgment: evidence in practice* (New York: Oxford University Press), 1–39.

Evidence-Based Medicine Working Group (1992), 'Evidence-based medicine: a new approach to teaching the practice of medicine', *Journal of the American Medical Association*, **268**: 2420–5.

Eysenck, H. (1991), 'Meta-analysis and its problems', *British Medical Journal*, **309**: 789–92.

Feinstein, A. R. and Horwitz, R. L. (1997), 'Problems in the "evidence" of evidence-based medicine', *American Journal of Medicine*, **103**: 529–35.

Gilbody, S. M. and Song, F. (2000), 'Publication bias and the integrity of psychiatry research', *Psychological Medicine*, **30**: 253–8.

Goodman, K. W. (2005), 'Ethics, evidence, and public policy', *Perspectives in Biology and Medicine*, **48**: 548–56.

Green, J. and Britten, N. (1998), 'Qualitative research and evidence based medicine', *British Medical Journal*, **316**: 1230–2.

Grossman, J. and Mackenzie, F. J. (2005), 'The randomized controlled trial: gold standard or merely standard?', *Perspectives in Biology and Medicine*, **48**: 516–34.

Guyatt, G., Rennie, D., Meade, M., and Cook, D. (2008) (eds.), *Users' guides to the medical literature: a manual for evidence-based clinical practice*, 2nd edn. (Chicago: AMA Press).

Haynes, R. B. (2002), 'What kind of evidence is it that evidence-based medicine advocates want health care providers and consumers to pay attention to?', *BMC Health Services Research*, **2** (3): 6 March <http://www.biomedcentral.com/1472-6963/2/3> accessed 27 January 2014.

Healy, D. (2001), 'Evidence-biased psychiatry?', *Psychiatric Bulletin*, **25**: 290–1.

Horwitz, R. I. (1996), 'The dark side of evidence-based medicine', *Cleveland Clinical Journal of Medicine*, **63**: 320–3.

Howick, J. (2011), *The philosophy of evidence-based medicine* (Chichester: Wiley-Blackwell).

Kelly Jr., R. E., Cohen, L. J., Semple, R. J., Bialer, P., Lau, A., Bodenheimer, A., Neustadter, E., Barenboim, A., and Galynker, I. I. (2006), 'Relationship between drug company funding and outcomes of clinical psychiatric research', *Psychological Medicine*, **36**: 1647–56.

Kerridge, I., Lowe, M., and Henry, D. (1998), 'Ethics and evidence-based medicine', *British Medical Journal*, **316**: 1151–3.

Kirsch, I., Deacon, B. J., Huedo-Medina, T. B., Scoboria, A., Moore, T. J., and Johnson, B. T. (2008), 'Initial severity and antidepressant benefits: a meta-analysis of data submitted to the Food and Drug Administration', *PLoS Medicine*, **5**: e45.

Knottnerus, J. A. and Dinant, G. J. (1997), 'Medicine based evidence a prerequisite for evidence based medicine', *British Medical Journal*, **315**: 1109–10.

Lam, R. W., Kennedy, S. H., Grigoriadis, S., McIntyre, R. S., Milev, R., Ramasubbu, R., Parikh, S. V., Patten, S. B., and Ravindran, A. V. (2009), 'Canadian Network for Mood and Anxiety Treatments (CANMAT) clinical guidelines for the management of major depressive disorder in adults. III. Pharmacotherapy', *Journal of Affective Disorders*, **117**: S26–S43. <http://www.canmat.org/resources/CANMAT%20Depression%20Guidelines%202009.pdf> accessed 24 February 2014.

Lau, J., Ioannidis, J. P. A., and Schmid, C. H. (1998), 'Summing up evidence: one answer is not always enough', *The Lancet*, **351**: 123–7.

Lexchin, J., Bero, L. A., Djulbegovic, B., and Clark, O. (2003), 'Pharmaceutical industry sponsorship and research outcome and quality: systematic review', *British Medical Journal*, **326**: 1167–70.

Malterud, K. (1995), 'The legitimacy of clinical knowledge: toward a medical epistemology embracing the art of medicine', *Theoretical Medicine*, **16**: 83–98.

Mathieu, S., Boutron, I., Moher, D., Altman, D. G., and Ravaud, P. (2009), 'Comparison of registered and published primary outcomes in randomized controlled trials', *Journal of the American Medical Association*, **302**: 977–84.

Miettinen, O. S. (1998), 'Evidence in medicine: invited commentary', *Canadian Medical Association Journal*, **158**: 215–21.

Miké, V. (1999), 'Outcomes research and the quality of health care: the beacon of an ethics of evidence', *Evaluation and the Health Professions*, **22**: 3–32.

Moher, D. (1993), 'Clinical-trial registration: a call for its implementation in Canada', *Canadian Medical Association Journal*, **149**: 1657–8.

Moncrieff, J. (2009), *The myth of the chemical cure* (New York: Palgrave MacMillan).

Moynihan, R., Heath, I., and Henry, D. (2002), 'Selling sickness: the pharmaceutical industry and disease-mongering', *British Medical Journal*, 324: 886–91.

Norman, G. R. (1999), 'Examining the assumptions of evidence-based medicine', *Journal of Evaluation in Clinical Practice*, 5: 139–47.

Oakley-Browne, M. A. (2001), 'EBM in practice: psychiatry', *Medical Journal of Australia*, 174: 403–4.

Perlis, R. H., Perlis, C. S., Wu, Y., Hwang, C., Joseph, M., and Nierenberg, A. A. (2005), 'Industry sponsorship and financial conflict of interest in the reporting of clinical trials in psychiatry', *American Journal of Psychiatry*, 162: 1957–60.

Polychronis, A., Miles, A., and Bentley, P. (1996), 'The protagonists of "evidence-based medicine": arrogant, seductive and controversial', *Journal of Evaluation in Clinical Practice*, 2: 9–12.

Ray, L. (1999), 'Evidence and outcomes: agendas, presuppositions and power', *Journal of Advanced Nursing*, 30: 1017–26.

Sackett, D. L., Rosenberg, W. M. C., Gray, J. A. M., Haynes, R. B., and Richardson, W. S. (1996), 'Evidence-based medicine: what it is and what it isn't', *British Medical Journal*, 312: 71–2.

Sackett, D. L., Richardson, W. S., Rosenberg, W., and Haynes, R. B. (1998) (eds.), *Evidence-based medicine: how to practice and teach EBM*, 1st edn., 8th printing (Edinburgh: Churchill Livingstone).

Sackett, D. L., Straus, S. E., Richardson, W. S., Rosenberg, W., and Haynes, R. B. (2000) (eds.), *Evidence-based medicine: how to practice and teach EBM*, 2nd edn. (Edinburgh: Churchill Livingstone).

Schott, G., Pachl, H., Limbach, U., Gundert-Remy, U., Lieb, K., and Ludwig, W. (2010), 'The financing of drug trials by pharmaceutical companies and its consequences', *Deutsches Ärzteblatt International*, 107: 295–301.

Sehon, S. R. and Stanley, D. E. (2003), 'A philosophical analysis of the evidence-based medicine debate', *BMC Health Services Research*, 3 (14): 21 July <http://www.biomed-central.com/1472-6963/3/14> accessed 28 January 2014.

Shahar, E. (1997), 'A Popperian perspective of the term "evidence-based medicine"', *Journal of Evaluation in Clinical Practice*, 3:109–16.

Sismondo, S. (2008), 'Pharmaceutical company funding and its consequences: a qualitative systematic review', *Contemporary Clinical Trials*, 29: 109–13.

Spielmans, G. I. and Parry, P. I. (2010), 'From evidence-based medicine to marketing-based medicine: evidence from internal industry documents', *Bioethical Inquiry*, 7: 13–29.

Straus. S. E. and McAlister, F. A. (2000), 'Evidence-based medicine: a commentary on common criticisms', *Canadian Medical Association Journal*, 163: 837–41.

Straus, S. E., Richardson, W. S., Glasziou, P., and Haynes, R. B. (2011) (eds.), *Evidence-based medicine: how to practice and teach EBM*, 4th edn. (Edinburgh: Elsevier Churchill Livingstone).

Tanenbaum, S. J. (1993), 'What physicians know', *New England Journal of Medicine*, 329: 1268–71.

Tonelli, M. R. (1998), 'The philosophical limits of evidence-based medicine', *Academic Medicine*, 73: 1234–40.

Tonelli, M. R. (2006), 'Integrating evidence into clinical practice: an alternative to evidence-based approaches', *Journal of Evaluation in Clinical Practice*, **12**: 248–56.

Tonelli, M. R. (2009), 'Evidence-free medicine: Forgoing evidence in clinical decision making', *Perspectives in Biology and Medicine*, **52**: 319–31.

Tonelli, M. R. (2012), 'Compellingness: assessing the practical relevance of clinical research results', *Journal of Evaluation in Clinical Practice*, **18**: 962–7.

Traynor, M. (1999), 'The problem of dissemination: evidence and ideology', *Nursing Inquiry*, **6**: 187–97.

Turner, E., Matthews, A. M., Linardatos, E., Tell, R. A., and Rosenthal, R. (2008), 'Selective publication of antidepressant trials and its influence on apparent efficacy', *New England Journal of Medicine*, **358**: 252–60.

Upshur, R. E. G. (1999), 'Priors and prejudices', *Theoretical Medicine and Bioethics*, **20**: 319–27.

Upshur, R. E. G. (2001), 'Meaning and measurement: an inclusive model of evidence in health care', *Journal of Evaluation in Clinical Practice*, 7:91–6.

Upshur, R. E. G. and Colak E. (2003), 'Argumentation and evidence', *Theoretical Medicine*, **24**: 283–93.

Urbach, P. (1993), 'The value of randomization and control in clinical trials', *Statistics in Medicine*, **12**: 1421–31.

Worrall, J. (2002), *What evidence in evidence-based medicine?*, ed. J. Reiss (Causality: metaphysics and methods, technical report 01/03; London: London School of Economics, Centre for Philosophy of Natural and Social Science) <http://www.lse.ac.uk/CPNSS/pdf/DP_withCover_Causality/CTR01-02-C.pdf> accessed 28 January 2014.

Worrall, J. (2004), *Why there's no cause to randomize*, ed. J. Reiss (Causality: metaphysics and methods, technical report 24/04; London: London School of Economics, Centre for Philosophy of Natural and Social Science) <http://www.lse.ac.uk/CPNSS/pdf/DP_with-Cover_Causality/CTR%2024-04-C.pdf> accessed 28 January 2014.

Worrall, J. (2010), 'Evidence: philosophy of science meets medicine', *Journal of Evaluation in Clinical Practice*, **16** (2010): 356–62.

Chapter 4

Psychiatry and evidence-based psychiatry

As is clear from the term, the concept of evidence-based medicine (EBM) is dependent on the more basic concept of medicine. What is meant by medicine is never discussed by EBM texts. Instead, medicine is taken to comprise certain tasks that doctors do: making diagnoses, offering prognoses and treatments, and monitoring potential harms. The original EBM authors were trained in the discipline of internal medicine, so it is not surprising to find that their reflections on the kinds of problems faced by clinicians—for which EBM was proposed as a solution—concerned this area of practice. These might include such questions as to what extent does a diagnostic test increase one's capacity to make a correct diagnosis; at what point in the course of a chronic condition (e.g. hypertension) should one intervene with treatment; and what are the advantages and disadvantages of intervening (i.e. of decreasing blood pressure)?

Whether the kinds of questions EBM was intended to address are of relevance to psychiatry is a question of central importance in the debate about the ethics of evidence-based psychiatry. Chapter 4 explores this issue, giving attention to some of psychiatry's assumptions about the nature of mental disorders and their treatments. Chapter 5 examines how psychiatric practice does, or does not, map on to evidence-based practice in light of these assumptions. An examination of the issues involved in applying EBM to psychiatry exposes some of the fault lines where ethical problems may emerge. Thus, Chapters 4 and 5 lay the foundation for an analysis of the ethics of evidence-based psychiatry.

The first section of this chapter discusses the evolution of the modern discipline of psychiatry and the assumptions about the nature of mind, disease, and treatment that are embedded within its practice. I attempt to define 'psychiatry', and in so doing show that the practice of psychiatry is framed by an unresolved debate about the nature of mind. Psychiatry, as a practical discipline, does not attempt to resolve this debate, even though various theoretical commitments are implied in its diagnoses and treatments. Section 4.2 defines evidence-based psychiatry and compares this definition to the views of the interviewees (see

Section 1.3 for details). The interviewees agreed that evidence-based psychiatry was defined by applying the rules of EBM to psychiatry, but believed it focused on applying evidence to psychiatric decision-making rather than integrating evidence with clinical expertise and patients' values, as described in the original model. Their main preoccupation was whether the evidence privileged by EBM is relevant to actual clinical decisions in psychiatry. In light of these views, Section 4.3 questions whether EBM can be applied to psychiatry, an issue taken up in more detail in Chapter 5.

4.1 What is Psychiatry?

4.1.1 Conceptual Commitments

Defining mental illness is the issue that has framed the entire field of psychiatry from its inception. It is important to acknowledge that psychiatry—or, perhaps more accurately, identifying and intervening in cases of madness—is a vast enterprise encompassing many transcultural and transtemporal histories. Some scholars believe there are aspects of mental disorders, such as specific symptoms like delusions, that are consistent regardless of culture or historical period. For example, using institutional records, some researchers have compared rates of certain mental symptoms during the nineteenth century with current rates (Beveridge 1995; Turner 1989). A key assumption behind this approach is that a symptom called by a certain name in the nineteenth century is the same entity referred to when we employ that term now. Whether this is the case or not is a matter of continued debate (Scull 1984); therefore, for our purposes, what constitutes a mental disorder requires demarcation by time period and geographical location. When I speak of psychiatry, I will be speaking of contemporary, mainstream, North American psychiatric practice.

The current standard textbook in North American psychiatry, *Kaplan and Sadock's comprehensive textbook of psychiatry* (Sadock et al. 2009), does not index a definition of psychiatry. However, the foreword begins with the following statement: 'Psychiatry is the medical specialty that diagnoses, treats, and cares for patients with mental or emotional disorders and related problems' (Michels 2009: lv). This seemingly straightforward definition is preceded by a rich history of the emergence of the concept of mental disorder, with its accompanying diagnoses and treatments, running in parallel with an equally complex story of how psychiatry became a medical specialty.

Although accounts of madness have been found dating back to antiquity, the eminent historian of medicine Roy Porter (2002) notes that, in Western thought, the distinct notion of a 'mental' disorder emerged only in the mid-eighteenth century. Prior to this time, non-religious theories of madness were somatic, meaning that they posited that certain derangements of bodily components (whether fluids such as humours or solids such as organs) led to states of madness. Inspired by contemporaneous philosophizing about the mind and how it worked, some scholars began to ascribe mad states to faulty mental mechanisms (though allowing that these faults may have been brought about by problems in bodily mechanisms). According to this view, there was some mental (that is, non-bodily) apparatus that must fail in order for madness to arise. However, since there was no distinct specialty of psychiatry at this time, general physicians were responsible for the investigation and classification of mad states, as well as the treatment and care of those thought to be mad (Porter 2002: 123–55).

In Western Europe, the next hundred years brought refinements in theorizing about the causality, classification, and treatment of mental disorders. The eventual success achieved by researchers in identifying anatomical or physiological changes associated with particular symptom clusters (e.g. spirochetes in the brains of those affected by general paresis of the insane) held promise for the elucidation of the biological causes—and the anatomical correlates—of all mental disorders.

Developments in the classification of mental disorders proceeded in tandem. Through careful clinical observation, disorders became distinguished from one another, particularly the disorders that were later classified as neurological, such as Parkinson's disease. New ideas about treatment emerged, including approaches such as social rehabilitation, then known as moral treatment. But there remained little success in curing insanity. This failure was particularly evident to the alienists—the doctors who supervised the growing network of public and private insane asylums. In spite of discouraging therapeutic results, they remained committed to treating the types of problems suffered by their patients. By the middle of the nineteenth century, alienists and researchers in several countries consolidated their authority by organizing themselves into specialist professional organizations with their own academic journals, while doctors secured state recognition of their expertise through medico-legal acts such as certification and involuntary hospitalization. By the early twentieth century psychiatry had emerged as its own medical specialty, with a distinct identity and specific training requirements (Porter 2002: 123–55).

By identifying itself as a branch of medicine, psychiatry implicitly committed itself to the theoretical commitments upheld by other branches of medicine (Reznek 1991: 13). Broadly, this theory is physicalist in that it views the world as containing only one kind of material—physical material—which is governed by the laws of nature. Human beings are part of the physical world and are therefore entirely physical themselves. Thus, human bodies are like complex machines, devoid of meaning and operating deterministically according to physical laws.

Kaplan and Sadock's comprehensive textbook of psychiatry (Sadock et al. 2009) provides various hints that contemporary Western psychiatry adheres to this physicalist view. For example, the foreword explains that the distinction between neurology and psychiatry does not lie in the organ of concern (the brain), nor does it lie in the 'nature of the underlying pathology or pathogenesis. . .' (Michels 2009: lvi).[1] The author assumes that the same types of pathologies encountered by neurologists—namely, specific anatomic or physiologic disruptions (strokes, haemorrhages, demyelinating conditions such as multiple sclerosis, genetic conditions such as Huntington's disease)—apply in psychiatry as well. Following the foreword, the first two chapters—which occupy 600 pages of the 4520-page textbook—are devoted to neuroscience and then neuropsychiatry and behavioural neurology (the psychiatric aspects of non-psychiatric conditions such as brain tumours, AIDS, headache, etc.).

Chapter 1 of *Kaplan and Sadock's comprehensive textbook of psychiatry* begins with the following statement: 'The human brain is responsible for our cognitive abilities, emotions and behaviours—that is, everything we think, feel, and do' (Grebb and Carlsson 2009: 1). This introductory section goes on to explain that the current method of psychiatric classification into symptomatically defined syndromes does not pick out 'discrete, biologically distinct entities', but that a brain-based—or at least a biologically based—diagnostic system would. It is within Chapter 3, in a section entitled 'Brain models of mind', that the book offers its sole indexed definition of mind. The text reads as follows:

> The word mind comes from minding, paying attention . . . and an ontologically neutral commonality that relates the material brain to minding has been identified: this commonality is 'information processing'. The ontological commonality is shown by a variety of conscious and unconscious processes that are coordinate with identifiable brain processes occurring in identifiable brain systems. By 'coordinate with' it is meant that at some level the descriptions of brain processes and descriptions of mental processes become homomorphic. An example from computer science illustrates what is meant by homomorphic: a word processor is used by typing English words and sentences. The word processing system, by virtue of an operating system using assembly language and say, ASCII, octal, or hexadecimal format, converts the keyboard input to binary, which is the 'language' of the computer. There is nothing in the description of English and that of binary machine language that appears to be similar . . . In a similar fashion, there is little in conscious experience that resembles the operations of the neural apparatus with which it has such a special relation. However, when the

---

[1] The author specifies that the difference between neurologic and psychiatric disorders lies in the skills required to provide optimal care and treatment.

transformations—the transfer functions, the codes that intervene between experience and neural operations—are sufficiently detailed, a level of description is reached in which the transformations of experience are homomorphic with the 'language' used by the brain . . . this language is the language of the operations of a microprocess taking place in synaptodendritic fields, a mathematical language similar to that which describes processes in micro- (i.e. subatomic) physics.

(Pribram 2009: 674)

According to this explanation, there is a direct correspondence between conscious mental activity and neurochemical activity in the brain. Furthermore, this citation adopts an explicit reductionist view by claiming that what is mental is fully explicable in physical terms. Yet this characterization does not actually explain how this correspondence takes place—that is, how ' . . . a mathematical language similar to that which describes processes in micro (i.e. subatomic) physics' equals a mental state. This problem is often referred to as the explanatory gap between the physical brain and conscious experience. To put it another way, tables are made of atoms but that does not mean that we will know everything we want to know about tables by studying atoms, nor can we necessarily talk about the characteristics that are important in tables (size, load-bearing capacity, finish, etc.) in the same language that we would use to talk about atoms.[2] Finding solutions to this problem remains an active area of debate in philosophy. However, the psychiatric description of 'mind', at least as represented in this passage, does not recognize the problem.

As Burwood and colleagues have argued (1999: 7–12), much of the ongoing debate in the philosophy of mind reflects a physicalist and, more precisely, a mechanical conception of body. If bodies really are physical entities operating mechanistically without meaning, this raises a series of questions about minds. Are minds physical entities like bodies or not? If minds are physical entities, then how do they give rise to psychological states? If minds are not physical entities, then what are they? How do minds cause physical things in the world, including in our bodies, to happen? Burwood and colleagues (1999) point out that the widely held mechanistic conception of body makes it difficult to imagine how mental life unfolds as it does. A view of bodies that is less mechanical and permits the integration between our physical and mental selves might not face the same philosophical bind. However, the mechanistic conception of body is accepted in medicine as unproblematic. Likewise, psychiatry endorses this physicalist conception of body and applies it equally to mind. Understanding the nature of what is mental is not an issue addressed

---

[2] The philosopher Ian Gold formulated the explanatory gap in this way.

directly by the field. Instead, a direct connection between physical events and mental states is simply assumed to be present.

4.1.2 Diagnosis and Treatment

The textbook definition of psychiatry provided earlier pointed to the field's two distinct but related tasks in determining: 1) what counts as a mental disorder and, by implication, how different disorders should be distinguished from each other (diagnosis and classification); and 2) how to intervene when we encounter someone who has a mental disorder (treatment).

4.1.2.1 *DSM* Definition

In North America, psychiatric disorders are defined and distinguished from each other according to the *Diagnostic and statistical manual of mental disorders (DSM)*,[3] currently in its fifth revision (*DSM-5*). The *DSM* is the accepted classification scheme by the mainstream of North American mental health professionals and is used widely in health care settings, within the legal system, and by insurance companies.

What is a mental disorder? The *DSM-5* defines it as:

> . . . a syndrome characterized by clinically significant disturbance in an individual's cognition, emotion regulation, or behavior that reflects a dysfunction in the psychological, biological, or developmental processes underlying mental functioning. Mental disorders are usually associated with significant distress or disability in social, occupation or other important activities. An expected or culturally approved response to a common stressor or loss, such as the death of a loved one, is not a mental disorder. Socially deviant behavior (e.g. political, religious, or sexual) and conflicts that are primarily between the individually and society are not mental disorders unless the deviance or conflict results from a dysfunction in the individual as described above.
>
> (American Psychiatric Association 2013: 20)

The *DSM-5* goes on to describe each individual disorder by listing its defining criteria and providing additional background information about its prevalence, course, familial pattern, and so on.

4.1.2.2 Causal Theory

While disease categories in medicine in general (including psychiatry) do not represent natural kinds in the philosophical sense (Reznek 1987: 63–79) (meaning that disease categories are constructed by humans rather than a reflection of what is found in nature), classification schemes of diseases should

---

[3] The International Classification of Diseases (ICD), produced by the World Health Organization, is also a widely accepted classificatory scheme, but is not commonly used within North America.

still allow clinicians to distinguish between different conditions. In other areas of medicine, pathogenesis helps to make these distinctions. Usually, a disease is classified according to its most basic known cause. In the case of infection, the most basic causal factor is the invading microorganism; hence, these conditions are classified as infectious diseases. In ischaemic heart disease, ischaemia is caused by narrowing of the coronary arteries, hence the term 'coronary heart disease'. Since the cause of the narrowed coronary arteries is complex, multifactorial, and not completely known, the disease state is classified by its most basic known cause: the narrowed coronary arteries.

Causal theory also underlies treatment. Ideally, medical treatment aims to intervene at the most basic level of causality that is known, which of course is determined by what the causal theory is in the first place. To return to the example of infection, antibiotics are designed to kill the causal agent—the invading bacteria. It would be insufficient to treat an infection only at a symptomatic level (e.g. treat an itchy skin infection with an antihistamine) if we know what the causal agent is and have the capacity to intervene at a more basic causal level than symptomatic control. Lung cancer is hypothesized to be caused (in part) by cigarette smoking. However, it is difficult to interrupt the causal process once a tumour has been discovered because the exposure to smoking has already taken place. Furthermore, the causal processes at the lung-tissue level are complex, multifactorial, and incompletely known (smoking is not the only relevant factor, since some smokers do not develop cancer and some people who develop lung cancer have never smoked). Thus, we intervene at the most basic pathogenetic level we do know—the level of tumour cells dividing. We aim to stop the cancerous tissue from propagating itself, growing larger, and causing more pulmonary dysfunction.

The conceptual allegiance between disease causality and treatment is perhaps best exemplified by fortuitous findings of successful treatment. If a treatment works there is a tendency to work backwards, assuming that the mechanism of an effective treatment must be interfering with the causal mechanisms of the disease. For example, the discovery that bright-light therapy seemed to improve depressive symptoms in people affected by seasonal affective disorder (major depression with a seasonal course, meaning onset of depression in late autumn or early winter and remission in spring) gave rise to the theory that this particular diagnostic entity was caused by lack of light[4] (Enns et al. 1999: 41).

Causal theory links diagnosis and treatment. If X causes condition Y, and treatment Z successfully interferes with X, condition Y can be cured or

---

[4] In fact, the cause of the disorder remains unknown.

improved using treatment Z. Knowing the cause and developing effective treatment are therefore directly connected. Treatments only aim for symptomatic relief when our causal theories are insufficiently developed to know what X is, or when our technologies are insufficiently developed to interfere with X. For example, patients with irritable bowel syndrome suffer chronically from a number of uncomfortable gastrointestinal symptoms, but why they experience these symptoms is unknown; therefore, the focus of treatment is reduction of the frequency and severity of the uncomfortable symptoms. We do know that various viruses cause the common cold, but we do not know how to eliminate the virus. Again, the only option is symptomatic relief.

The fourth edition of the *DSM* (*DSM-IV*) states that the term mental disorder '. . . should not be taken to imply that there is any fundamental distinction between mental disorders and general medical conditions[5] . . .' (American Psychiatric Association 1994: xxv). If this is the case, then the link between diagnosis, treatment, and causal theory in psychiatry should be similar to that for other medical disorders.

4.1.2.3 Theoretical Neutrality

From its third revision onwards, the *DSM* has developed a descriptive approach that has '. . . attempted to be neutral with respect to theories of etiology' (American Psychiatric Association 1994: xviii). Further, both *DSM-IV* and *DSM-5* contend that 'a diagnosis does not carry any necessary implications regarding the causes of the individual's mental disorder . . .' (American Psychiatric Association 1994: xxiii; 2013: 25). Note that the *DSM* does not try to liberate itself from theory but merely tries to be neutral between the various possible causal theories which, according to the definition of mental disorder, could be psychological, biological, or developmental. However, philosophers have questioned the idea that observations, such as *DSM*-descriptive criteria, can be theory neutral (Stanford 2009). How might theory play a role in descriptions of specific mental disorders?

Many of the criteria sets contain behaviours as possible signs of the disorder. Including behaviours as part of the definition of the disorder implies a belief in behaviourist theories of mind. This is clearer when we consider a

---

[5] The phrase 'general medical condition' is used in the *DSM-IV* to denote non-psychiatric conditions. For example, to diagnosis a psychotic disorder brought about by a brain disease such as a tumour, one would diagnose a 'psychotic disorder due to a general medical condition', where the general medical condition was the brain tumour. *DSM-5* drops the terminology 'general medical condition' altogether and substitutes it with 'other medical condition', which makes clear that the authors views psychiatric and medical conditions to be continuous.

comparison to a non-psychiatric disorder that—similar to psychiatric disorders—is diagnosed on the basis of self-reported symptoms and for which the pathophysiology is not well known, such as migraine headache. The criteria for the diagnosis of migraine headache do not include behaviours that might accompany a headache, such as clutching one's head or saying 'ow'. Why not? Because these behaviours, if they occur, are considered merely the consequence of the physiological dysfunction underlying migraine headache. In other words, behaviours are not part of the causal theory of migraine headache.

By contrast, the disruptive, impulse control, and conduct disorders are centred on difficulties in self-control of behaviours (and emotions) (American Psychiatric Association 2013: 461). Problems in behaviour constitute the disorder, rather than the behaviours merely being the result of an underlying dysfunction. For these types of mental disorders, our behaviours define what is mental. The diagnosis of conversion disorder offers another different example. A patient with conversion disorder experiences 'one or more symptoms of altered voluntary motor or sensory function' (American Psychiatric Association 2013: 318). If the person is feigning or inducing these symptoms for the purpose of appearing sick, he will be diagnosed with a factitious disorder and, if it is for the purpose of obtaining some other benefit (e.g. disability insurance payments), he will be diagnosed with malingering. In other words, by definition, the patient must not be aware of bringing on these symptoms, yet the symptoms are not explained by another medical condition. The definition of this disorder demonstrates its commitment to a notion of the unconscious as part of the theory of mind operating within this definition.

Thus, the *DSM* is not theoretically neutral with respect to etiology, but rather theoretically plural, with various theories embedded in different diagnoses. Reznek has argued that, as a field, psychiatry incorporates a variety of theories of mental disorder—psychodynamic, biological, cognitive, behavioural, sociological, and intentional (1991: 145–56)—which can operate singly or in combination in describing causes of mental disorders. In fact, *DSM-5*'s authors acknowledge that the manual '. . . must be applicable in a wide diversity of contexts . . . by clinicians and researchers of many different orientations (e.g. biological, psychodynamic, cognitive, behavioral, interpersonal, family/systems)' (American Psychiatric Association 2013: xli). The word 'orientations' hides the fact that these are theories—some independent of each other, some working in concert. This plethora of theoretical orientations reflects the absence of an agreed-upon theory of mind within the field of psychiatry, even in the face of psychiatry's implied acceptance of physicalist theories of body and brain.

4.1.2.4 **Theoretical Pluralism**

Theoretical pluralism is also evident in the variety of available psychiatric treatments. These treatments can broadly be grouped as psychological (psychotherapy—with individuals, couples, families, or groups) and biological (medications, electroconvulsive therapy, transcranial magnetic stimulation, deep brain stimulation, and psychosurgery). Biological treatments are informed by physicalist theory, meaning that they are thought to work by inducing biochemical and neurophysiological (neurotransmitter) changes in the brain, which necessarily bring about changes in conscious experience. By contrast, psychotherapies operate at experiential and intersubjective levels. How exactly these therapies bring about changes to mental states is a matter of debate. One view is that psychotherapies work as medications do: by altering the brain physically through its neurochemical processes (Gabbard 1994: 16), which then changes one's conscious experience.

A contrary view is that one cannot think about psychological change in biochemical terms because psychological terms cannot be reduced to biological ones; thus, any theory of psychological change must be expressed in psychological terms such as having a 'corrective emotional experience' (Yalom 1995: 24–8). Certain therapies, such as cognitive therapy, have developed their own mid-level theory of change (related to the way that people process information), which can then be related to brain functioning. In general, when a treatment is successful in improving the symptoms of a mental disorder, an assumption is often made that the treatment's mechanism of action is related to the etiological pathway of the disorder. But because several different types of interventions (medications, different types of therapy) seem to be effective in changing mental states, theoretical pluralism in psychiatric therapeutics has flourished, and psychiatry's capacity to resolve questions of etiology remains as limited as that of philosophy.

As a medical discipline, psychiatry's ultimate aim is effective healing. The pragmatic impulses of medicine steer psychiatry away from an unresolved philosophical debate about minds and ambivalence about its own underlying theories towards practical concerns of how to intervene when someone experiences troublesome mental states, however they are defined. It is here that EBM has provided an ideal companion to psychiatry. Psychiatric disorders lack known pathophysiology. Randomized controlled trials (RCTs) can be used to test the effectiveness of treatments even in the absence of known pathophysiology. In fact, according to EBM, pathophysiologic rationale is not considered an adequate or even necessary basis to determine whether treatments are effective. In this respect, the field of psychiatry is particularly well suited to adopt

EBM, because psychiatrists are not tied to, and therefore not as reluctant to give up, the kinds of pathophysiological explanations of disease and treatment mechanisms well established in other medical specialties.

Furthermore, EBM offers psychiatrists an opportunity to make claims about treatment effectiveness without having to understand what causes mental disorders and without having to address thorny philosophical questions about the nature of its subject matter. Ashcroft has argued that EBM can be applied without a uniform theory of causation and explanation (2004: 134). This helps psychiatry to establish its scientific credibility, even in the absence of an established body of pathophysiologic knowledge. The next section defines evidence-based psychiatry and explores how this marriage of EBM and psychiatry works in practice.

4.2 What is Evidence-based Psychiatry?

4.2.1 Defining Evidence-based Psychiatry

Since its original description in 1990, EBM has received a great deal of attention from psychiatrists. However, unlike EBM, there is no official text that describes evidence-based psychiatry.[6] This raises the question of who is entitled to speak for evidence-based psychiatry and define its terms. There are, for example, psychiatrists who work in evidence-based psychiatry units (Gray and Pinson 2003), edit evidence-based mental health journals,[7] and teach EBM to psychiatry trainees (Agrawal et al. 2008); however, the extent to which these individuals share a common understanding of evidence-based psychiatry is unknown. In the absence of an agreed definitive source for evidence-based psychiatry, it is reasonable to infer that it is simply the straightforward application of the definition and rules of EBM to psychiatric practice (Geddes and Harrison 1997; Goldner and Bilsker 1995; Goldner et al. 2001; Gray and Pinson 2003). Thus, any attempt to understand evidence-based psychiatry is really an attempt to understand EBM and how well it applies to psychiatry.

As in EBM, the concept of evidence is central to evidence-based psychiatry. There is no definition of evidence that is specific to psychiatry, but its meaning can be inferred from the evidence hierarchy. Geddes and Harrison (1997)

---

[6] Although, three psychologists have developed a handbook entitled *Clinicians' guide to evidence-based practices: mental health and the addictions* (Norcross et al. 2008), which describes evidence-based practice for psychologists. On its back cover, it is endorsed by a psychiatrist as well as a social worker, who praises its applicability to all mental health practice.

[7] See, for example, the journal *Evidence-Based Mental Health*.

lay out an evidence hierarchy specifically for studies of psychiatric treatments, since therapeutics is the area in which the majority of psychiatric clinical research studies are undertaken. This hierarchy is very similar to the evidence hierarchy described in Section 2.1.6. The similarity between these two hierarchies further demonstrates that evidence-based psychiatry results from the direct application of EBM to psychiatry.

> Evidence from a meta-analysis of RCTs
> Evidence from at least one RCT
> Evidence from at least one controlled study without randomization
> Evidence from at least one other type of quasi-experimental study
> Evidence from non-experimental descriptive studies, such as comparative studies, correlation studies and case-control studies
> Evidence from expert committee reports or opinions and/or clinical experience of respected authorities
>
> (Geddes and Harrison 1997)

From this hierarchy, we can infer that psychiatric evidence is quantitative data drawn from experimental studies, preferably RCTs or meta-analyses of such trials. These authors provide no further specification of evidence.

Evidence-based psychiatry's emphasis on empirical quantitative data stands in contrast to actual patient encounters in clinical psychiatry. Unlike most medical specialties, in which data obtained in the clinical encounter mostly comprises measurements of various types (whether through physical examination techniques or the results of laboratory or imaging investigations), the standard patient encounter in psychiatry resembles a qualitative research interview—oral, in-depth, exploratory, and individualized. While the interview is structured by the psychiatrist's diagnostic and therapeutic aims, interviewers are expected to weave together the information that their patients provide into an evolving picture of the whole person. Thus, the skilled psychiatrist has both quantitative and qualitative aims. Quantitatively, she enumerates patients' symptoms and evaluates their severity, using them to classify each patient as an example of a more general (diagnostic) category. Qualitatively, she elucidates the patient's individual personal narrative and contributes to its evolution and meaningfulness. The evidence hierarchy aims to substantiate beliefs and decisions regarding the quantitative (nomothetic) aspects of clinical psychiatry but is silent about the qualitative (idiographic) dimension of the psychiatrist's work.

4.2.2 The Five Steps of EBM Revisited

The five steps of EBM remain unchanged for evidence-based psychiatry. But do these steps apply to psychiatry? Recall that the first three steps involve formulating questions that arise in clinical care in the PICO format; using electronic databases to identify research articles or summaries that address the question; and then using the critical appraisal questions to judge the quality of the articles (see Section 2.2). Some types of clinical questions in psychiatry may be amenable to this process, such as those that involve choosing medications for treatments upon the first evaluation of a single and specific disorder. However, there are a great many problems in clinical practice that are not amenable to this approach at all. Some examples of common, but difficult, clinical challenges include how to treat patients with problems that do not fit into specific diagnostic categories; how to handle any of the numerous therapeutic impasses (frequent missed appointments, lack of participation, self-defeating behaviours) that arise in treatment; and how to interpret and respond to strong feelings towards a patient (either positive or negative). In such cases, the best evidence is found on the lowest rung of the hierarchy, the 'clinical experience of respected authorities'—often one's colleagues.

The situation is somewhat different when one arrives at step 4, and must take evidence and integrate it with patients' biology, values, and preferences. This involves answering the integration questions (see Figure 2.1) outlined in Chapter 2: 1) Is our patient so different from those in the study that its results cannot apply? 2) Is the treatment feasible in our setting? 3) What are our patient's potential benefits and harms from the therapy? 4) What are our patient's values and expectations for both the outcome we are trying to prevent and the treatment we are offering? The first question—Is our patient so different from those in the study that its results cannot apply?—is difficult to answer, as individual psychological differences make it very challenging to predict whether a strategy is likely to apply. In other words, even if a patient does fit within a larger diagnostic category (e.g. people with major depressive disorder), individual psychological characteristics will influence how a treatment is adopted and takes effect, perhaps even more so than whatever characteristics he shares in common with other patients who have the same diagnosis. For any given patient, the relative importance of individual differences versus shared characteristics is difficult to determine. In reality, it is the answers to questions 2–4 that will guide practice. For example something that is not feasible cannot be provided, regardless of the evidence or the values of the patient. Something that runs counter to a patient's values will either not be tried or not be accepted, regardless of the evidence or feasibility (unless it is imposed).

Looking at the five steps in action, it appears that evidence-based psychiatry in real practice situations will mostly involve taking the suggestions of colleagues and seeing which of these can be implemented and accepted by patients. Put this way, the question is not whether EBM applies to psychiatry, but rather whether these steps offer anything different from what existed pre-EBM. If they do, then the difference must lie in something other than following the five steps as described in the EBM texts.

In their guide to evidence-based practice in psychology, Norcross and colleagues (2008) apply EBM to clinical psychology. The EBM approach is largely unchanged in their application, with one important difference:[8] the authors are clear that in evidence-based psychological practice, evidence, clinical expertise, and patients' values and preferences (or what they call 'patients' characteristics, culture, and preferences') are not equal. Research data takes priority over the other elements and is the starting point for decision-making (Norcross et al. 2008: 5). Using case examples, Norcross and colleagues explain that evidence-based interventions should always be employed unless: 1) the patient, through the process of informed consent, refuses; 2) the patient has tried all available evidence-based therapies but they have failed; or 3) there is a compelling reason (related to internal or external validity) why the evidence-based intervention does not apply to the patient.

Applying EBM to psychology changes practice to favour interventions supported by RCTs unless there is a specific, mitigating reason to do otherwise, whereas applying EBM to psychiatry seems to result in practice that is not greatly different from what existed before. Which of these options most closely resembles evidence-based psychiatry in action? The views of the EBM experts I interviewed help to shed light on this question.

4.2.3 What is Evidence-based Psychiatry, According to the Experts?

At the beginning of this chapter I noted that the emergence of psychiatry was accompanied by an implicit commitment by the field to the theories underlying the rest of medicine and by a demand for recognition as a specific area of medical expertise. In the present era, evidence-based psychiatry reinforces this connection between psychiatry and the rest of medicine. As one participant said:

> 2-10: 'There is a specific problem for mental health care because psychiatry throughout its history, modern psychiatry since the Enlightenment, has always been characterized by huge struggles, and one of them was a desperate struggle to be part of medicine. And to share the income, the status, and all that of the rest of medicine. And maybe

---

[8] There are other minor differences, but privileging research evidence is the most substantial theoretical difference.

our patients have benefited from that to some extent. I'm not saying that's good or bad but that's very much one of the hard problems of psychiatry . . . And for that, evidence-based medicine was sent from heaven because now we've got something. We can produce trials as well, and yes, we can do that just like you, we are also good medics and proper medics more importantly.'

According to this view, evidence-based psychiatry's primary contribution has been to fill an important social role in the evolution of psychiatry as a profession and as a branch of medicine. However, most other participants focused on the role of EBM in psychiatric practice and the extent to which it could be used in that domain. Participants from the EBM developer group tended to believe that the basic principles of EBM could be applied to research and practice in psychiatry.

> I: 'Do you think evidence-based psychiatry is any different from that [EBM] or is it pretty much the same thing, but just applied to psychiatry?'
> 1-8: 'If it is different, I have no idea how or why. It seems like it should be exactly the same thing.'

However, they worried that decisional incapacity among psychiatric patients would make it harder to have the kind of shared decision-making process described in the EBM texts. The other two groups of interviewees saw evidence-based psychiatry differently, viewing it as an approach to psychiatric practice that prioritized evidence (rather than clinical expertise and patients' values) in clinical decision-making. They then questioned whether this evidence could be straightforwardly applied to most psychiatric decisions. At least one participant did not think that there was anything particular about psychiatry that made the application of EBM problematic, but rather believed that the application of EBM to any specialty had problems because its basic principles were flawed.

> 3-12: 'I've yet to find a group that claims this as their own really because even the people in clinical practice, who you'd think would be the ones that would say "well EBM was for us", don't think it's for them. They think it was an epidemiological thing foisted on them and now they're stuck trying to figure out how to apply this to an individual patient . . . It's got these epidemiological underpinnings but at the same time it really was geared toward clinical practice but in an inappropriate way because it really doesn't help physicians to figure out how to balance all these different sources of evidence, and values, and everything else and make that clinical decision . . . I'm sure that advocates of EBM would think that you could just transfer it right across [to psychiatry]. I'd say no, you can't just take the principles of EBM and apply them to evidence-based psychiatry, and just use them in psychiatry but that's not because there's something unique in psychiatry so much as that the principles themselves were already problematic in the first place.'

Some interviewees noted that psychiatrists, more so than other types of physicians, have to pay more attention to patient and context-specific factors in clinical decision-making. The following quotation implies that choices about drugs may be amenable to the EBM approach, whereas other areas of practice, such as discharge-planning, may not be because the population orientation of EBM may not apply to the individual nature of these types of decisions.

> 1-9: 'So a lot of the management plans in psychiatry seem to be heavily influenced by plausible options for the patient, determined by life circumstances, emotional psychological reserve, social supports, the environment in which the person lives. And that makes perfect sense . . . That's the exposure that I have to psychiatry and, in the context of what we've been talking about, it [psychiatric decision-making] does seem highly appropriately context-, and patient-, and setting-specific.'

Interviewees who worked in the domain of mental health tended to believe that evidence (rather than clinical expertise and patients' values) was the defining feature of EBM. Their main concern was about the amount and quality of research data that psychiatrists had to draw upon.

> 2-6: '. . . so in mental health there's less evidence . . . there's less empirical evidence out there so there's still a role for my judgement and experience and whatever to play in the context of making a clinical decision. The principles are the same. The dataset is smaller.'

The viewpoints expressed by the two preceding interviewees are distinct in an important way. The first (1-9) suggests that there are areas of psychiatric practice that necessarily rely on individualized assessment through clinician expertise (or experience), and are simply not amenable to group-level experimentation. Therefore, there may be many clinical decisions for which evidence of the type favoured by EBM cannot apply. These types of decisions will not be 'evidence-based' in the sense of being supported by highly ranked forms of data. However, such decisions may still be rational and defensible. The second view (2-6) suggests that there is a type of inverse relationship between evidence and expertise. If there is an abundance of data on a topic, there is less of a role for expertise. As the body of empirical data expands, the need for expertise and/or experience necessarily diminishes. Both views stand in contrast to the view promoted by EBM's authors, in which EBM applies regardless of the type of decision being made, and where the three elements of evidence, expertise, and patients' values operate for all clinical decisions.

4.3 **Does EBM Apply to Psychiatry?**

4.3.1 **Diagnosis in Psychiatry**

Many interviewees thought that the nature of mental disorders and their treatments meant that they could not easily be investigated using the EBM approach. For example, some participants observed that the nature of psychiatric diagnosis is different from diagnoses in other areas of medicine. Because the research methods listed on the evidence hierarchy are dependent on diagnosis, this makes a direct application of EBM more problematic. The first quotation below alludes to the difficulty of comparing individuals with the same diagnoses, let alone groups of people who have the same diagnosis, while the second suggests that some psychiatric diagnoses are more stable and precise than others. Where there is greater precision, EBM applies.

> 2-7: 'The problem is that diagnoses in psychiatry are much more fluctuating. They are not stable, and they are much more a matter of definition. So they are not natural entities. And so this again makes it difficult to compare cases, even if they have the same diagnosis.'

> 3-11: '. . . an example of an area where an evidence-based approach was appropriate is in the treatment of depression because severe depression, major depression, is a condition where at least some of the complexities I'm talking about are lost. It's a bit more like having appendicitis than, say, a personality disorder. So it's a condition where the effect of different approaches to treatment could be looked at in a traditional evidence-based way to good effect.'

Another participant expressed the concern that basing clinical research on diagnosis was problematic in psychiatry compared to other areas of medicine because diagnosis and prognosis in psychiatry were insufficiently correlative. In other words, if one reason to do clinical trials is to determine which treatments improve health for a given condition, one must first know the prognosis of that condition in order to know when to intervene and what one is attempting to achieve by intervening. If psychiatric diagnosis does not correlate well with prognosis, then even high-quality evidence of treatment effectiveness will not help to make longer-term predictions about when, for how long, or even whether to intervene.

> 2-2: 'One of the ways in which evidence-based psychiatry is fundamentally different to evidence-based medicine is that in evidence-based practice as we have it . . . the currency in which we categorize patients and their needs and on which we base our interventions is diagnosis . . . Having a psychiatric diagnosis A versus psychiatric diagnosis B tells you very, very little about the future history of a patient's condition, and in particular their future need for care compared to people with the next category.'

The two quotations below hone in on the perennial problem of diagnostic validity. In the absence of an objective standard of verification (such as an abnormal lab result, physical exam sign, or imaging finding) how can we establish what any specific disorder is and who is affected? The second quotation also speaks to the problem of manipulation or dishonesty in light of the validity problem. If a disorder cannot be verified, its boundaries and/or defining characteristics can be modified. Therefore, what constitutes successful treatment can vary according to the desires of researchers or clinicians. In commenting on the 'abuse of evidence-based medicine' the second interviewee refers to the potential for pharmaceutical companies and their investigators to expand diagnostic categories in order to enlarge markets for their products, and then to define therapeutic improvement in such a manner that the experimental treatment is likely to be successful.

> 3-13: 'Diagnosis in psychiatry is very different than it is in other areas of medicine, since it relies on self-report or on report of behavioural patterns or experiences.'

> 2-4: '. . . there's a tremendous amount of mistrust over psychiatric syndromes. Because not only can we select the outcomes . . . we can uniquely manufacture outcomes. We could also manufacture scales custom to the application. So I think psychiatry is more prone to the abuse of evidence-based medicine.'

These interviewees underline the concern that for EBM to apply diagnoses need to be valid, stable, and prognostically predictive, and that this may not be the case for psychiatric diagnoses. These participants have framed the problem of applying EBM to psychiatry as one in which the assumptions embedded within EBM as to the nature of disease may not fit with the nature of psychiatric disorders.

4.3.2 **Treatments in Psychiatry**

Several participants suggested that complex interventions commonly used in psychiatry, such as psychotherapy or social rehabilitation, are difficult to evaluate using EBM-preferred research methods because of the challenge in specifying every element of the intervention and carrying them all through in clinical trials and into clinical practice. Furthermore, the outcomes that these interventions are trying to effect may be more difficult to measure than 'hard' endpoints (such as death) in medicine or surgery.

> 3-5: 'On the face of it, it should be a simple deductive inference that if medicine and psychiatry are continuous, then evidence-based medicine and evidence-based psychiatry should be continuous, conceptually. But there is the question of whether evidence-based psychiatry and psychiatry are continuous, because people will say that what is evidence-based psychiatry does not map onto psychiatrists' accounts of what

they're doing, or patients' accounts of what they're doing in the following sense: that the kinds of things that you can test using the sorts of methodology favoured by EBM are actually not typical of the majority of things that psychiatrists do, or want to do, for their patients. And the sort of outcomes that you can measure in such tests are not the sort of outcomes that psychiatrists want to influence or their patients want to have influenced.'

2-4: 'The outcome is not as easy to operationalize as outcomes in hypertension; for example, heart attack or death or stroke. Ultimately, in psychiatry the objective could be viewed as living the good life. What is it to live a good life or to live well, and what's a life worth living even? And regardless of depression scores . . . we're dealing with increasingly distant proxies to the good life.'

These participants' concerns highlight the difficulties in drawing a strict parallel between the experimental evaluation of a drug and its target outcome in, say, cardiology, versus a social or psychological intervention in psychiatry. First, as discussed in Section 4.3.1, there are problems in defining the study groups using psychiatric diagnosis, given their instability and imprecision. It is unclear to what extent groups of patients sharing diagnoses are truly similar, and whether they can be straightforwardly compared with similar diagnostic groups in other studies. Second, there is the difficulty in specifying the outcome. What are psychiatrists trying to achieve in treating their patients? Reductions in symptom levels, which tend to be the outcome of interest in most therapeutic effectiveness research in psychiatry, may or may not correlate particularly well with quality of life, well-being, or flourishing. This stands in contrast to an outcome such as a reduction in blood pressure, which does correlate with a reduction in risk of stroke and hence with potential enhancement to quality of life. Third, there are problems in specifying the intervention. A drug's chemical composition can be precisely characterized, while the elements and dynamic interactions within a complex intervention such as a housing support programme cannot.

In fact, EBM is necessarily committed to an active ingredient concept—that is, the notion that an effective treatment contains an active ingredient that has some specific action in the sick body. This commitment explains EBM's prioritization of the RCT, a research method considered most able to isolate the effect of the active ingredient. It also favours the view that the important thing to measure is changes in illness-specific features, such as changes to psychiatric symptom-rating scales,[9] because this is where an active ingredient will

---

[9] Psychiatric clinical trials will often assess before and after scores of symptom-rating scales as a measure of change during the trial. Examples of commonly used scales include the Hamilton Rating Scale for depression (HAM-D) and the Positive and Negative Symptoms Scale for Schizophrenia (PANSS).

have its direct action. The active ingredient concept reinforces the notion that effective treatments represent specific technologies rather than composite, interacting, elements (such as the so-called, non-specific therapeutic factors of psychotherapy).

Notwithstanding these conceptual matters, there are practical considerations. Even if an intervention is effective according to the standards of EBM, and the evaluation truly captures how the intervention is used in practice, it might be difficult to offer it in practice if it is complex and requires considerable time to learn. This is a greater problem for psychotherapy-practising psychiatrists than for those who restrict their work to prescribing medication.

> 2-5: '. . . if you as a psychiatrist were trained primarily in pharmacology and you read that the best treatment for depression is CBT [cognitive behavioural therapy] but you haven't had any training in CBT, what are you going to do? Your choices are either, "well, let me shut down my practice for three months and go off somewhere and get training in CBT, or not see these patients, which is a lucrative part of my income, or continue doing what I have been doing". Guess what the average practitioner is going to do? So I think the impact of EBM is limited to interventions that are easy to implement.'

Participant 2-5 implies that EBM favours pharmacological treatments in psychiatry because it is this style of practice in which changes are easier to implement. What does this mean for the future of treatments and practitioners who use different approaches? This issue is considered further in Chapter 5.

4.4 **Conclusions**

Chapter 4 has tried to define evidence-based psychiatry. Given the absence of a specific text or acknowledged authority on this point, I have tried to understand evidence-based psychiatry by reference to its two parent concepts: EBM (discussed in Chapter 2) and psychiatry. Psychiatry has inherited the legacy of a philosophical debate concerning the nature of minds. In concerning itself with the suffering brought about by problems in thinking, feeling, and behaving, psychiatrists have not necessarily tried to resolve this debate but have focused their energies on the practical matters of trying to address the problems that are brought to them. Of course they cannot avoid the debate and, in determining the scope of their field and their expertise, they necessarily offer various responses to the question of what constitutes a mental disorder and, by extension, a mind. These various responses demonstrate the plurality of theories—sometimes complementary, sometimes opposing—that underscore the practice of psychiatry.

EBM has offered more than just a pragmatic approach to the usual business of practising psychiatry. Because it carries certain assumptions about the nature of disease and treatment, adopting EBM pushes psychiatry to accept these assumptions. Are these assumptions correct? Many of the EBM experts I interviewed raised concerns that they are not. The next chapter develops this theme in greater detail, considering the various issues that arise in the application of EBM to psychiatry.

References

Ashcroft, R. E. (2004), 'Current epistemological problems in evidence-based medicine', *Journal of Medical Ethics*, 30: 131–5.

Agrawal, S., Szatmari, P., and Hanson, M. (2008), 'Teaching evidence-based psychiatry: integrating and aligning the formal and hidden curricula', *Academic Psychiatry*, 32: 6.

American Psychiatric Association (1994), *Diagnostic and statistical manual of mental disorders*, 4th edn. [*DSM-IV*] (Washington: APA Press).

American Psychiatric Association (2013), *Diagnostic and statistical manual of mental disorders*, 5th edn. [*DSM-5*] (Arlington, VA: APA Press).

Beveridge, A. (1995), 'Madness in Victorian Edinburgh: a study of patients admitted to the Royal Edinburgh Asylum under Thomas Clouston, 1873–1908 (part I)', *History of Psychiatry*, vi: 22–54.

Burwood, S., Gilbert, P., and Lennon, K. (1999), *Philosophy of mind* (Montreal: McGill-Queen's University Press.)

Enns, M. W., Levitan, R. D., Levitt, A. J., Dalton, E. J., and Lam, R. W. (1999), 'Diagnosis, epidemiology, and pathophysiology', in Lam, R. W. and Levitt, A. J. (eds.), *Canadian consensus guidelines for the treatment of seasonal affective disorder* (Vancouver: Clinical & Academic Publishing), 20–63.

Gabbard, G. O. (1994), 'Basic principles of dynamic psychiatry', in: *Psychodynamic psychiatry in clinical practice*, 2nd edn. (Washington: American Psychiatric Publishing Incorporated), 3–28.

Geddes, J. R. and Harrison, P. J. (1997), 'Closing the gap between research and practice', *British Journal of Psychiatry*, 171: 220–5.

Goldner, E. M., and Bilsker, D. (1995), 'Evidence-based psychiatry', *Canadian Journal of Psychiatry*, 40: 97–101.

Goldner, E. M., Abbass, A., Leverette, J. S., and Haslam, D. R. (2001), 'Evidence-based psychiatric practice: implications for education and continuing professional development', *Canadian Journal of Psychiatry*, 46: 15 pages following p. 424.

Gray, G. E. and Pinson, L. A. (2003), 'Evidence-based medicine and psychiatric practice', *Psychiatric Quarterly*, 74: 387–99.

Grebb, J. A. and Carlsson, A. (2009), 'Introduction and considerations for a brain-based diagnostic system in psychiatry', in: Sadock, B. J., Sadock V. A., and Ruiz, P. (eds.), *Kaplan and Sadock's comprehensive textbook of psychiatry*, 9th edn. (Philadelphia: Lippincott, Williams and Wilkins), 1–5.

Michels, R. (2009), 'Foreword: the future of psychiatry', in: Sadock, B. J., Sadock V. A., and Ruiz, P. (eds.), *Kaplan and Sadock's comprehensive textbook of psychiatry*, 9th edn. (Philadelphia: Lippincott, Williams and Wilkins), lv-lix.

Norcross, J. C., Hogan, T. P., and Koocher, G. P. (2008), *Clinician's guide to evidence-based practices: mental health and the addictions* (New York: Oxford University Press).

Porter, R. (2002), *Madness: a brief history* (Oxford: Oxford University Press.

Pribram, K. H. (2009), 'Brain models of mind', in: Sadock, B. J., Sadock V. A., and Ruiz, P. (eds.), *Kaplan and Sadock's comprehensive textbook of psychiatry*, 9th edn. (Philadelphia: Lippincott, Williams and Wilkins), 674–83.

Reznek, L. (1987), *The nature of disease* (London: Routledge and Kegan Paul).

Reznek, L. (1991), *The philosophical defence of psychiatry* (London: Routledge).

Sadock, B. J., Sadock, V. A., and Ruiz, P. (eds.) (2009), *Kaplan and Sadock's comprehensive textbook of psychiatry*, 9th edn. (Philadelphia: Lippincott, Williams and Wilkin).

Scull, A. (1984), 'Was insanity increasing? A response to Edward Hare', *British Journal of Psychiatry*, 144: 432–6.

Stanford, K. (2009) 'Underdetermination of scientific theory', *The Stanford Encyclopedia of Philosophy* (Winter 2009 edn.), ed. E. N. Zalta <http://plato.stanford.edu/archives/win2009/entries/scientific-underdetermination/> accessed 26 June 2013.

Turner, T. (1989), 'Rich and mad in Victorian England', *Psychological Medicine*, 19: 29–44.

Yalom, I. D. (1995), 'Interpersonal learning', in: *The theory and practice of group psychotherapy*, 4th edn. (New York: Basic Books), 17–46.

Chapter 5

The critique of evidence-based psychiatry

5.1 The Critical Literature Concerning Evidence-based Psychiatry

2-9: 'But of course in psychiatry, particularly, hearing these terrible stories from the past from giving malaria to patients and all sorts of horrible things which had been done in the name of treatment, makes EBM particularly important.'

Among the mental health practitioners I interviewed for this book, several believed that evidence-based medicine (EBM) is the best way of safeguarding psychiatry and psychiatric patients from unproven fads or dangerous interventions. They pointed out that the history of psychiatry is littered with failed interventions but that EBM could prevent this problem from recurring in the future. If something really works, EBM will tell us. Patients will no longer have to fear that they would be subject to unproven therapies as they had been in the past. This way of conceiving the role of EBM within psychiatry links it to an ethical aim: to safeguard patients from harm that might otherwise occur without the use of these methods. Whether EBM can achieve this goal depends on whether it can provide the knowledge that will lead to improved health or, at least, less harm. Most of the debate about evidence-based psychiatry has revolved around this concern.

The critiques of evidence-based psychiatry challenge EBM to varying degrees. Some authors argue that while EBM makes sense in theory, it fails in practice because the type of knowledge it provides is difficult to apply to real clinical problems in psychiatry. Others go further, arguing that while EBM applies well to evaluating pharmaceuticals, it cannot readily be applied to other types of interventions such as psychotherapy, or complex interventions such as supported housing programmes or assertive community treatment. Still stronger is the claim that psychiatric disorders and their treatments simply do not conform to EBM's underlying assumptions about the nature of disease and treatment; thus, EBM cannot be applied to any psychiatric treatments. In this section, I examine each of these positions in turn.

5.1.1 **EBM is Sound but its Implementation is not**

This critique takes the position that, while the principles of EBM are sound, EBM-preferred research studies do not reflect actual psychiatric problems and patients sufficiently for the results to be clinically useful (Seeman 2001). For example, patients enrolled in randomized controlled trials (RCTs) in psychiatry usually have one specific problem (e.g. depression), unlike patients in real practice who often have several problems (e.g. depression comorbid with anxiety symptoms and substance abuse). Thus, it is unclear to what extent RCT data obtained by studying patients with a single problem can be applied to patients with multiple problems. Another example is that follow-up in research studies, particularly RCTs of pharmaceutical agents, is often short-term (weeks); however, the actual treatment of mental disorders is usually long-term (years), as these disorders are in most cases chronic or relapsing and remitting (Oakley-Browne 2001). According to Healy (2001), this mismatch between the parameters of clinical trials of pharmaceuticals and the realities of actual patients' problems results from the fact that the majority of clinical trials are designed for a business purpose—to achieve regulatory approval and thus market access—rather than a scientific or clinical one.

Regulators, such as the Center for Drug Evaluation and Research (CDER) of the US Food and Drug Administration, require that a drug can be shown to be safe and efficacious in at least two adequate and well-controlled studies (US Food and Drug Administration 2013). These studies are then subject to internal review. In the words of the CDER:

> Drug companies seeking to sell a drug in the United States must first test it. The company then sends CDER the evidence from these tests to prove the drug is safe and effective for its intended use. A team of CDER physicians, statisticians, chemists, pharmacologists, and other scientists reviews the company's data and proposed labeling. If this independent and unbiased review establishes that a drug's health benefits outweigh its known risks, the drug is approved for sale.
>
> (US Food and Drug Administration 2011)

While this approach incorporates standards of good clinical research, it is first and foremost a threshold for what can be safely and honestly sold in the marketplace. The assessment of the balance between health risks and benefits in terms of what should be approved for sale might be quite different from the risk–benefit assessment made by a patient with a specific medical problem, or even by a group of patients with the same problem. For example, both the CDER and the Therapeutic Products Directorate of Health Canada (which performs the same function in Canada as the CDER does in the US) state that drugs destined for chronic use need to demonstrate their rates of adverse events for 6–12 months (Center for Drug Evaluation and Research 1988; Health Canada 1995). While they argue that most adverse events are likely to be identified in this time-frame, a patient who is being recommended a medication for long-term use, as is often the case in psychiatry, might consider a 6–12-month timeframe to be too short. For example, the antipsychotic drug olanzapine has been associated with weight gain and dyslipidemia. While these effects are likely to appear within the first 12 months of treatment (Pérez-Iglesias et al. 2014), the development of their sequelae—such as type 2 diabetes mellitus—may take much longer. In order to accurately estimate the risk of these sequelae, studies would need to be longer.

In spite of these concerns, for some authors EBM could be applied to psychiatry provided research studies matched psychiatric patients and problems more closely. Countering this claim, Welsby (1999) argues that for many patients the interactions between multiple medical conditions and multiple interventions over time represents a state of complexity that EBM-preferred research methods can never capture. Take, for example, a typical population of patients from a psychiatric clinic servicing disadvantaged people who have depressive symptoms, occasional substance abuse and regular alcohol consumption, while at the same time being unemployed. Some of these people will attend AA erratically, participate in community centre activities, and/or work with social services personnel at a primary-care health centre. These activities may all have therapeutic potential and may interact differentially with symptoms of depression and/or with substance use: participation in AA may help to eliminate alcohol consumption for some participants, which may simultaneously increase feelings of depression due to reflection about one's past behaviour.

Now imagine that we try to conduct an RCT of antidepressant therapy involving this group. Even if one could define a homogenous population of such patients in terms of their multiple diagnoses or symptom clusters, it does not seem feasible for an RCT to take into account the interaction between these and the different potentially therapeutic (or harmful) interactions at play over time. RCTs may be very good at establishing the efficacy of single interventions in diagnostically homogenous populations, but in psychiatry these situations are the exception rather than the rule; thus, it is hard to know how one could apply the knowledge that RCTs might be good at providing to populations that are diagnostically and therapeutically different.

5.1.2 **EBM Applies to Studies of Psychiatric Medication but not Psychotherapy or Other Non-pharmacological Interventions**

Proponents of this argument claim that the narrative structure and meaningfulness of personal experience are essential components of living with a mental disorder and, in particular, the psychotherapeutic treatment of mental disorders. Mental states are complex, subjective experiences and these may be resistant to measurement, at least in the manner envisioned by EBM (Holmes 2000). For EBM to work, the subject under investigation (whether a mental state or a treatment) must be clearly defined, its components must be identifiable and separable from the background circumstances, and its effects must be measurable discretely—ideally quantitatively—in order that statistical testing can then be applied to the measurements. Pharmacological treatments have specific biological characteristics and effects that can be defined, measured, and thus controlled for in RCTs. By contrast, what patients experience when they suffer from a mental disorder and/or during psychotherapeutic treatment cannot necessarily be reduced to discrete biological or quantitative terms. As a result, EBM cannot be applied neatly to the investigation of psychotherapeutic and social interventions. For Holmes (2000), this should not lead to the abandonment of research of non-psychopharmacological interventions but is rather a call to refine alternative research methods. It is also a plea for evidence-based psychiatry to construe research and evidence more broadly, in order to include difficult-to-research phenomena such as subjective and intersubjective experiences. These might include the hows and whys of patient experiences of 'feeling understood', or a particular desire felt by clinicians to 'go the extra mile' for certain patients (Bohart et al. 1998).

The challenges involved in evaluating psychotherapy offer an example of the potential problems of applying EBM to research of non-pharmaceutical interventions. If researchers choose the highest-ranked method on the evidence hierarchy, the RCT, they will have difficulty fulfilling several of the criteria for high-quality research identified by EBM. Recall that EBM's critical appraisal process involves answering three questions: 1) Are the results valid? 2) What are the results (what is the size of the effect)? and 3) How can I apply these results to patient care (or to a specific patient)? The first question concerns the internal validity of the study: the degree to which a study can yield truthful conclusions about the question it is trying to answer. The third question contained four components, the first being the extent to which the study participants are comparable to one's own patients and, therefore, the extent to which study results can apply to one's patients. This is a question about external validity, which is the degree to which a study's conclusions can be generalized beyond the conditions of a study to some broader situation. In the case of clinical trials, these would be conclusions that extend beyond the specific trial participants to a larger group of patients.

5.1.2.1 Internal Validity

Achieving a high degree of internal validity can be particularly difficult in RCTs of psychotherapy and other complex interventions in mental health. For example, blinding of the patient may be quite difficult to achieve, even if the control condition is a placebo therapy (meaning something that is structured like a real course of psychotherapy without the specific technical elements being tested). In testing psychological treatments, it is unlikely that patients will be unaware whether they are receiving an actual therapy or a control condition, particularly if the consent process has been properly undertaken.

The study therapists will certainly know which condition they are offering. The researchers who assess change in the patients might be blind at the start, but it may be difficult to remain blind throughout the assessment process if both patient and therapist know to which groups they were assigned.[1] Difficulties in blinding lead to the kinds of biases EBM's authors worry about, such as patients who know they are receiving a therapy trying harder to get better, or reporting that they are better compared with those receiving the control condition. Establishing and maintaining an appropriate control condition is another problem for psychotherapy research. Because a great many things that may be therapeutic are not considered to be treatments—visits with friends, improved employment prospects, increased revenue—it is very difficult to establish that the control group is not receiving 'therapies' that have similar effects as the study treatment. In fact, McMahon has argued that it may simply be difficult to achieve good controls in psychiatric research (2002: 1367).

5.1.2.2 External Validity

Achieving a high degree of external validity may also be a challenge in psychotherapy research. For example, how should a therapy be delivered in a research study such that the findings of the study will map onto how the therapy is delivered, given the institutional and resource constraints in real clinical practice settings? There are major differences between a pill that can be self-administered in seconds and psychotherapy—a dynamic, interpersonal

---

[1] Fisher and Greenberg (1993) argue that even in drug trials of psychotropic medications, maintaining the double-blind is very difficult. Participants and researchers are often able to figure out the assignment.

interaction that evolves over much longer periods of time, the precise details of whose implementation are personality dependent and unique to every dyad. If the therapy is of the same duration as it often is in actual practice, it is likely to be so long that there will be a large number of dropouts from the study, and/or treatment effects will be confounded by patients' use of other interventions (e.g. reading self-help books, religious participation, etc.). A related problem involves defining the intervention under investigation. Again, it is more difficult to isolate the active ingredient in a psychotherapy compared to an active ingredient in a pill. In clinical practice, the therapist might utilize a variety of psychotherapeutic techniques within the same course of treatment, rather than a pure form of any one therapy. Even in a study where the therapeutic intervention is closely described—often in manual form—the research therapists may bring different qualities to the treatment being offered that the study participants may find particularly helpful or particularly harmful. These might include the therapist's voice or body language, or the memories that the therapist stirs up in the participant.

Offering a relatively shorter, purer course of treatment (meaning the study therapists abide strictly by therapy manuals and/or scripts) might avoid these methodological problems, and is the approach currently adopted by much psychotherapy research held up as evidence-based. This raises two questions. First, can something like psychotherapy be made pure, meaning that the only active ingredient is the technique? Second, even if it is possible, will studying a therapy this way be externally valid: will it provide results that are generalizable to longer-term clinical practice? The pure manual-based, standardized intervention offered in such trials is not typical of what the vast majority of patients are able to access through local health services. Thus, there is a question of whether these trials are testing interventions that can be delivered in practice.

5.1.2.3 Alternative Approaches

One possible solution to the problems of trying to conduct RCTs of psychotherapy is to conduct pragmatic trials. Pragmatic trials emulate real world conditions—in this case, the conditions of real clinical practice in terms of eligibility criteria, duration of the intervention, and type of intervention (Roland and Torgerson 1998)—compared to an explanatory trial, in which the goal is to determine whether an intervention can do what it is supposed to be able to do (for which one requires the precise conditions under which the effect should happen). A pragmatic trial might include a greater diversity of patients and exclude fewer of them than a typical explanatory trial, or there might be compromises to strict randomization. The US-based National

Institute of Mental Health (NIMH)-funded STAR*D trial (Clinicaltrials.gov 2009) was an example of such a trial. It investigated the effectiveness of certain antidepressants among a broad group of patients over several phases of treatment: initial trial, combination therapy, switching, etc. In STAR*D patients were offered choices of treatments at different study phases. For example, those patients who did not achieve remission of depression after the first trial of an antidepressant could choose either switching to a different medication or adding a different medication. Those who chose to switch would be randomized to one of three medication choices, but the initial choice to switch was theirs.

Another possible approach to evaluating psychotherapy in a way that might preserve its meaningfulness, to use Holmes' (2000) words, is for researchers is to employ alternatives to clinical trials such as one of various qualitative approaches. However, it is not clear how results from this type of research would be evaluated according to the rules of EBM, or if they would be counted at all. *Users' guides* includes a chapter on critically appraising qualitative research (Giacomini and Cook 2008: 341–60), but qualitative research is not included on the evidence hierarchy for studies of treatment. This suggests that treatments cannot or should not be studied in this manner.

The point here is that the nature of psychotherapy as an intervention is such that, whether one tries to investigate it using pragmatic designs, qualitative methods, or even a strict RCT design, the studies will necessarily be less internally valid than efficacy trials of pharmaceutical agents; thus, the data will perpetually lack the same degree of credibility. As a result, adhering to EBM may have the effect of marginalizing certain types of interventions, particularly those that are the most challenging to break down into discrete components, because they will never have the best support from the highest-ranked methods. In their comprehensive review of psychotherapy research, Roth and Fonagy address this problem when they write: '. . . while we can see that the absence of evidence of efficacy cannot and must not be equated with absence of evidence of effectiveness, this scientific review can only draw conclusions from the evidence available (1996: 34).

To what extent does marginalization actually occur in evidence-based psychiatry? The journal *Evidence-Based Mental Health*, which adheres to EBM principles, summarizes 'the highest quality original and review articles' (Evidence-Based Mental Health 2012: 30). In 2012, all the original and review articles of psychotherapies included in the journal used an RCT design, which is actually a journal requirement. The blinding varied. Most used blind assessors of outcome, while participants were mostly not blinded.

In other words, for their work to be considered of the highest quality, psychotherapy researchers must adhere to the evidence hierarchy as much as possible. If they do so, their studies will not be marginalized, in the sense that they could potentially be included in EBM resources alongside studies of pharmaceuticals. But whether adherence to EBM in research will translate into equal acceptability of psychotherapy compared to pharmaceuticals in clinical practice is unknown.

5.1.2.4 Evidence-based Psychology

Scholars within psychology are actively engaged in debate about whether the nature of psychotherapy itself makes it difficult to study. In their book *Evidence-based practices in mental health: debate and dialogue on the fundamental questions*, Norcross and colleagues (2006) invited numerous academic psychologists to debate the key issues involved in the application of the principles of EBM to psychotherapy research. The format of the book invited exchange: position papers on key questions were followed by responses. On the question of 'what qualifies as research on which to judge effective practice', the authors by and large accepted methodological pluralism as a necessary means of advancing knowledge of psychotherapy effectiveness. They included several methods not mentioned on the evidence hierarchy, such as case studies, qualitative research, and change process research (Norcross et al. 2006: 57–130). Other authors were equally pluralistic about the appropriate subjects of enquiry for psychotherapy research. In addition to the modality or technique of therapy, they tended to agree that the therapist, the patient, and the relationship between the two were necessary ingredients of effective therapy and required study. The debates in this book hint at the notion that evidence-based psychology may evolve into a broader approach to evaluating the effectiveness of psychotherapeutic interventions than evidence-based psychiatry. However, whether the robust pluralism envisaged by the authors will actually come to fruition is another question that remains unanswered.

Despite the fact that psychotherapy and other complex mental health interventions prove difficult to study using a strict EBM framework, the arguments discussed thus far accept that the effectiveness of pharmacological treatments for psychiatric disorders can be studied relatively unproblematically in accordance with the rules of EBM. In the next section I argue that the nature of psychiatric disorders is such that the rules of EBM, particularly the criteria for high-quality research, are not applicable.

5.2 Does EBM Apply to Psychiatric Disorders and their Treatments?

The rules of EBM make certain assumptions about disease and treatment. The first is that a diagnosis is a relatively precise definition that classifies the patient into a uniform group of patients with various shared characteristics, including clinical presentation and prognosis. This assumption is of fundamental importance because before one can conduct any kind of research study of an intervention, regardless of its place on the hierarchy, one has to assemble prognostically homogeneous patient groups. This is necessary to meet EBM's criteria for validity. Without prognostically homogenous groups one cannot draw conclusions about the efficacy of the interventions being tested, since it will always be plausible that the prognostic mix in the study groups influenced the results.

A second assumption of EBM's highly ranked research methods is that treatment effects can be defined by discrete changes and measured quantitatively. Recall that the second of EBM's three key critical appraisal questions is: 'What are results (what is the size of the effect)?' This question shows that a key function of the rules of EBM is to represent the size of intervention effects in quantitative terms. Broader effects or outcomes, such as improved quality of life or enhanced well-being, can be captured by breaking them down into smaller measurable units. Therefore, a related assumption is that measuring these smaller units will accurately reflect the larger category from which they are derived. This section explores whether these assumptions hold in researching psychiatric disorders.

5.2.1 Prognostic Homogeneity

In *Evidence-based medicine*, one of the basic critical appraisal criteria by which to evaluate studies of treatments is whether '. . . the groups were similar in all prognostically important ways at the start of the trial' (Straus et al. 2011: 172). Homogeneity of this type involves having similarities in severity of disease, overall health status, and sociodemographic factors that are presumed to be relevant to outcome.

5.2.1.1 Combinations of Diagnostic Criteria

Some authors raise the question of whether prognostic homogeneity can actually be achieved for psychiatric disorders (Maier 2006; Gupta 2007). In psychiatric practice, sets of diagnostic criteria create descriptions of clinical syndromes that enable psychiatrists to diagnose mental disorders and distinguish among them. The *Diagnostic and statistical manual of mental disorders*

(*DSM*) used by North American psychiatrists is a compendium of these sets for various diagnostic categories (American Psychiatric Association 2013). Each category is defined by a list of criteria, a minimum number of which must be met for a patient to be classified as belonging in a particular diagnostic category (e.g. there are nine possible criteria for major depression: a patient must have at least five of them, including depressed mood or loss of interest or pleasure, in order to be diagnosed as depressed). Inherent to the way that psychiatric diagnoses are made is the heterogeneity in clinical presentations of patients. One patient may have five of nine criteria for major depression, while the next patient may also have five criteria but only three of these might overlap with the first person's criteria. In fact, there are 70 possible combinations of four symptoms that someone with major depression might possess (assuming each combination includes one of the required symptoms). Then there are also patients who have six, seven, eight, or all nine symptoms. There are 93 possible combinations of these numbers of symptoms (again assuming each combination includes one of the required symptoms, except in cases of all nine symptoms in which the person has both required symptoms). Furthermore, within each uniform symptom group, each symptom or combination of symptoms may vary in severity from another person with that same combination. Are all of these different combinations of number, not to mention differential severity of symptoms, prognostically similar?

5.2.1.2 Within-Category Variability

The current division of major depression into melancholic and atypical subtypes is a real example of symptom differences leading to within-category prognostic variability. People with the atypical subtype of major depression experience some symptom reversal compared to patients with the melancholic subtype (i.e. weight increase instead of loss, hypersomnia rather than insomnia). Atypically depressed patients may respond better to different types of medications than melancholic patients (Lam et al. 2009). However, if the two groups were assumed to be prognostically similar because all patients shared several symptoms of major depression, and were mixed together in a clinical trial of a treatment, the results might not be helpful in guiding practice for either group. This example seems to suggest that it is possible to answer empirically whether specific combinations of symptoms with specific degrees of severity are prognostically similar or different from other combinations. One could assemble groups with certain combinations of symptoms at particular degrees of severity, and then follow them over time in order to evaluate whether they are prognostically similar to groups with other combinations of symptoms or with differing degrees of severity.

Given the enormous number of subgroups this would entail, this approach may not be feasible. Notwithstanding feasibility, there is another conceptual problem in trying to achieve prognostic homogeneity: unique or unusual symptoms.

5.2.1.3 Unique or Unusual Symptoms

A person might have all or almost all the criteria needed to be diagnosed with a disorder, yet also have unique or unusual symptoms that are not included on the list. How much flexibility should there be in interpreting whether an idiosyncratic symptom conforms to one described in the *DSM*? For example, upon being asked to describe her mood in words, one of my patients said: 'I feel dead'. I asked her what the feeling state 'dead' represented, and offered various mood descriptors (sadness, despair, hopelessness) but the best way she could describe her state was to say she feels 'dead'. Assuming she had at least four additional criteria of major depression, a researcher would have to decide whether 'feeling dead' can be reasonably interpreted as the equivalent to feeling depressed or some other symptom. Some assessors in this situation might conclude that feeling dead is the equivalent of feeling depressed and others might not. Including such people in a patient group of major depressives in a clinical trial may mean including patients who actually have a different disorder altogether that shares some features with major depression. Alternatively, excluding such patients might mean losing important clinical information about a distinct subtype of major depressives—those who feel dead.

5.2.1.4 Heterogeneity

Differences among patients unaccounted for by existing diagnostic criteria have the potential to lead to substantial heterogeneity within apparently uniform diagnostic groups. These differences could have a major impact on research data concerning prognosis, comorbidity, and treatment. In other areas of medicine, diagnostic features are usually measurable by methods external to the patient and the doctor. There may well be some degree of interpretation about the severity or even the presence of some physical signs, but most physicians have some forms of measurement at their disposal such as laboratory tests, imaging results, and so on. For example, a patient with abdominal pain could have various diseases. In determining which it is, it helps the physician to know whether inflammation was visible in the colon during colonoscopy. The presence of inflammation would enable the doctor to correlate the patient's pain with certain disease states and not others. However, for the patient who feels dead, the psychiatrist must make a determination of whether her reported subjective state does or does not correlate with a symptom (depressed mood), and whether her whole clinical presentation correlates with a disorder (major depression), without the assistance of any other measurement.

These interpretive difficulties between doctor and patient are compounded by the further problem of inter-patient differences in interpretation of symptoms. As the word 'depression' becomes increasingly common in lay discourse, it takes on diverse meanings. What one person means by depression or depressed mood may not be what another person means. Thus, both patient and assessor must engage in a considerable degree of interpretation, even when making a diagnosis using explicit criteria. The variability in clinical presentation (including both the symptoms themselves and their severity), along with these interpretive differences, means that it is not possible to ensure prognostic homogeneity, even within a single diagnostic group.

5.2.1.5 Randomization

But won't randomization solve this problem? Randomization achieves prognostic homogeneity by evenly distributing unknown confounding variables across diagnostic groups that are otherwise uniform. For psychiatric disorders, in which different patients may have different combinations of symptoms at different degrees of severity, one may not be starting with a uniform group to randomize. The randomization process will not change this fact. Moreover, Worrall (2002) has argued that randomization can only evenly distribute unknown confounders with indefinite replications of a clinical trial, but clinical trials are not repeated indefinitely; rather, they are conducted only once. Thus, it is possible that in any given trial one or more unknown confounders are distributed unevenly between trial groups.

What are the implications of this problem for RCT data in psychiatry? At the very least, even without taking this problem into consideration, RCT data will continue to represent heterogeneous populations and psychiatrists will continue to misapply these data to individual patients in practice without making potentially important clinical distinctions among subgroups. One possible solution to this lack of uniformity at the starting point is to assemble patient groups along one symptom (e.g. suicidal thinking) rather than one disorder. In this way, randomization would apply to all other symptoms, in treating them as potential confounders. This might be a useful approach when one wants to answer a research question about a specific symptom, such as how many people with suicidal thinking make an attempt. However, it would not be able to say anything about the broader syndromes. Another approach would be to assemble patient groups who did have exactly the same combinations of symptoms. While this adheres more closely to the assumptions of EBM, the results of such studies may or may not apply to patients with other combinations of symptoms.

5.2.2 **Quantification of Outcomes**

A second important assumption behind EBM-preferred research is that the outcomes of medical interventions can be, and should be, measured quantitatively. The evidence hierarchy for treatment makes clear that quantitative data resulting from RCTs or meta-analyses of these trials achieves the highest rating of validity of research designs. In evidence-based psychiatry, psychiatric outcomes—specifically changes in symptoms in response to a given treatment—are usually quantified using symptom-rating scales. Can symptom-rating scales reveal changes in the psychological states of people with mental disorders? If so, do these scores tell us what we want to know about the interventions under study? Do rating scale scores reflect those aspects of disorders that are most important to patients?

5.2.2.1 Weighing Outcomes

Specific symptoms may have more or less importance for a given patient. For example, in measuring changes in depressive symptoms, someone might report that her appetite has improved and yet she might still feel terribly depressed. Assuming that this person finds depressed mood a more troubling symptom than disruption in appetite, should her change in appetite weigh less heavily into her final score on a symptom-rating scale than the persistence of her depressed mood? Schaffer et al. (2002) have demonstrated that patients find the burden of suffering associated with some symptoms greater than with others. In response, rating scales can be designed to weigh certain symptoms more heavily than others. However, any weighting system may not be applicable to a given patient who rates the burden of suffering differently from the way in which the scale is designed. Thus, a final score will not necessarily reveal the burden of suffering relevant to any individual person. Defenders of quantification may respond that the point of such measurements, and of trials in general, is not to evaluate individual suffering but rather the average suffering or improvement in the study population. However, in order for the average result to be useful, its component parts—the individual scores of individual study participants—must accurately reflect their experiences.

5.2.2.2 Representing Meaning

Quantitative outcome measures also raise the more basic questions of whether numerical representations of experience can convey meaning. For example, one of my patients described the two prior episodes of depression he had experienced. When I asked him to rate his mood during these episodes using a rating scale of 0–10 (0 representing severe depression and 10 representing no depression), he rated his mood when at its worst during both episodes as 1 out of 10. However, he described these episodes as being completely different experiences, unequal in any way apart from the rating. Over the course of treatment, I asked this patient to rate the change in his mood on the same 0–10 scale; he said that his mood improved from 5 out of 10 to 7 out of 10 in a recent period. What does this tell us? We know his mood changed and that he was feeling somewhat better, but it is unclear if the change of two units tells us anything beyond the qualitative description 'better'. Is the difference between 5 and 6 equal to, or different from, the difference between 6 and 7? Defining change in numerical terms may falsely impose the logic of numbers onto subjective experience and create a false sense of knowledge about the extent, value, and importance of the experiential change to the patient.

Goldenberg (2006) has argued that a scientific account of disease may be of limited relevance to patients whose experience of illness has little to do with objective change and more to do with changes in the relationship between themselves, their embodiment, and the world. Psychiatric practice—and psychotherapy in particular— takes these experiential aspects of illness into consideration, but Goldenberg argues that research should also reflect this perspective (2006: 2629–30).

5.2.2.3 The Experience of Disorder

To some extent, everyone's experience of illness is unique, however much one shares in common with another sufferer. This is as true in coronary artery disease as it is in schizophrenia. Where psychiatric disorders differ from most other disorders is that, according to our current state of knowledge, the experience of the disorder is the disorder. Most other disorders have this subjective, experiential component as well as a biological component, which is understood in greater or lesser detail depending on the disorder. Table 5.1 illustrates this difference.

Table 5.1 Subjective versus objective aspects of disease

Disease examples	Fracture	Hypertension	Mental disorders	Schizoid personality disorder?
Objective aspect	yes	yes	no	no
Subjective aspect	yes	no	yes	no

A fracture, for example, frequently presents subjectively with pain in the affected area, and can be correlated by an objective measurement on an x-ray. Hypertension may cause no change in experience to its sufferers but can be measured using a blood pressure apparatus. Mental disorders lack this type of objective correlation: there is only the change to one's experience of one's life. In fact, a small minority of psychiatric disorders lack even this subjective experiential change. Sufferers are not necessarily distressed by their psycho-pathological states, although these states may lead to social or occupational impairment.

In general, medical treatment aims to modify the person's subjective experi-ence of disease through modification of the objective (usually biological) vari-ables. But in spite of whatever knowledge we have about the biological basis of psychiatry, at this point we cannot definitively draw specific pathophysiologi-cal or psychopathological conclusions about mental disorders. Patients and providers are left to diagnose and treat mental disorders at the level of expe-rience rather than by intervening with known biological variables. Another example from major depressive disorder illustrates this point. A patient reports that he has interrupted sleep as part of his depression. Poor sleep is a vegetative symptom (Akiskal 2009: 1701) and is considered to be biologically mediated, compared to psychological symptoms such as sadness and guilt. Treatment would not be considered successful unless these psychological symptoms of depression improved. If these symptoms improved but his sleep never returned to normal this would be unfortunate, but would not lead to the conclusion that his treatment had been a failure. Psychiatric treatments aim to target sub-jective experiences, not merely biological symptoms; in clinical practice, the subjective experience of wellness is more important clinically than changes in biological indices.

5.2.3 Technical Bias

The challenges of studying mental disorders and their treatments point to the issue of the technical bias of the evidence hierarchy. Recall that technical bias refers to our tendency to measure what we know how to measure using exist-ing methods or techniques, thereby reinforcing our knowledge of and belief in the importance of the phenomena we can investigate. Various phenomena that are central to psychiatric practice would be impossible to investigate using EBM's highly ranked methods. These include third party testimony (collat-eral history), the clinician's subjective feelings in response to a patient, and intersubjective experiences such as complicated dynamics enacted between psychiatrist and patient. All these phenomena are used in clinical practice as diagnostic evidence or as evidence when evaluating treatment effects. But because very little effort has been invested in researching their clinical value, they remain marginal from the point of view of being evidence-based. One will not find clinical guidelines in psychiatry that discuss how and when psychiatrists should, or should not, use their emotional reactions towards patients as diagnostic criteria. If we attempted to study these phenomena we would have to accept methods that are either low-ranked or unranked according to the evidence hierarchy. The problem is that, according to the principles of EBM, such research—and the phenomena it investigates—will always be considered tentative and of lesser scientific value compared with phenomena investigated by the highest-ranked methods. Thus, the technical bias of the evidence hierarchy privileges certain kinds of knowledge in psychiatry over others. What is the clinical value of these other phenomena? If we adhere to the evidence hierarchy, we will not find out. The worry is that technical bias unduly constrains psychiatric knowledge and, as a result, clinical care. The practising psychiatrist is left with a dilemma: adhere to the relatively narrow range of practices vetted by EBM-preferred research and evidence-based guidelines or draw upon practices that are little studied or studied only by low-ranked or unranked methods.

Faulkner and Thomas (2002) offer another perspective on the problem of technical bias by pointing out that mental health system users are typically not involved in the research planning process. These authors locate the 'technical' bias in the preoccupations of the researchers rather than in the methods per se. Researchers develop methods that measure those things they think are important. Meanwhile, the authors believe that users ought to lead the development and execution of research studies because user-led studies are more likely to focus upon questions and outcomes important to users, rather than those considered important by psychiatric researchers adhering to the demands of evidence-based psychiatry. They cite a study designed by users that 'explores people's strategies for living and coping with mental distress'. This qualitative study concluded that, according to service users, self-help and peer support were important strategies in learning to live with a mental disorder, particularly in overcoming stigma and discrimination. These issues, and the methods needed to study them, may not receive attention in the absence of user involvement in research, reinforcing the belief that what it is important to know about mental disorder derives solely from the questions that academic researchers can and want to answer.

In Chapter 3 we saw that those most expert in evidence-based psychiatry believe that EBM can be applied straightforwardly to psychiatric disorders and their treatments. In this chapter, we have questioned this belief, looking at three particular aspects of EBM in action (prognostic homogeneity, quantification of outcomes, and technical bias). Does adherence to EBM help us to distinguish the interventions that really work from unproven fads, thereby strengthening the ethics of practice, or does it marginalize topics we need to know about in order to practise psychiatry well? Depending on our answer to this question, EBM may or may not be a better guide to practice than what preceded it.

5.3 Pursuit of the Active Ingredient

5.3.1 Specific Deficit-Active Ingredient

Chapter 4 discussed the importance of the 'active ingredient' concept in EBM. The assumption that treatments exert a positive effect by virtue of an active ingredient lies at the heart of EBM and its prioritization of the double-blind RCT, a method whose strength lies in its ability to isolate the effect of an active ingredient on a disease process by controlling for the effects of other influences. The active ingredient concept reflects a particular view of therapeutic efficacy, whose applicability to mental disorders and their treatments is discussed in this section.

The active ingredient concept includes four elements. The first is that health problems can be broken down into specific, discrete components. For example, a fractured leg bone is a health problem with several components: the bone fracture disrupts the normal function of the leg; the person will be less physically mobile but may still have to get around, so some method of ambulation has to be found; the leg may have to be immobilized in order to heal but this process itself may lead to certain consequences such as skin breakdown or compression of nerves; surrounding tissues, which will have to be treated, may have been damaged at the time of the fracture; and pain and swelling caused by the fracture may be disruptive in terms of physical function and may also affect quality of life. The second element is that treatments will improve health problems by effecting change on one or more of these component parts; thus, for example, the broken leg is to be treated by providing an active ingredient for each component: a cast for the fracture, crutches for mobility aids, and painkillers for pain. The third element is that the perceptions, feelings, and attitudes a person has when he experiences a health problem—unless they are caused physiologically by the disease—are not part of the problem itself but are something like a reaction to it. For example, specific types of brain tumours may produce psychotic symptoms; therefore, these symptoms would be considered part of the original problem. By contrast, childhood traumatic experiences that are triggered when a person undergoes a colectomy for ulcerative colitis as an adult would be considered a reaction to the problem rather than part of the problem. The fourth element is that improvement in a problem's component parts will lead to improvements in subjective well-being; thus, treating each part with active ingredients is what is required for successful treatment, and the inverse also applies—that therapeutic success can be attributed to active ingredients working on component parts.

A medical problem is conceptualized as one in which there is a specific deficit (e.g. lack of insulin in type 1 diabetes), failure (e.g. decreased capacity for the heart to pump blood in congestive heart failure), or abnormality (e.g. the presence and growth of cancerous cells) that a successful treatment will target in order to reverse the problem, or at least correct it as well as possible. Advances in medical knowledge frequently relate to characterizing with ever-greater precision the nature of the deficit that underlies a given disease and the development of more specific treatments to target these deficits. EBM can thus play a role in determining whether the interventions we develop to identify and treat these deficits are effective in doing so.

The question here is whether this portrayal of disease actually fits with what we know about psychiatric disorders and their treatments. There are competing theories of the psychological deficits involved in mental disorders, and there are psychological therapies that target these deficits, based on the underlying theory of the origin of the deficit. However, to date, psychotherapy researchers have found comparable effectiveness among all therapies, regardless of their underlying theory (Wampold 2013: 21; Wampold et al. 1997). In his landmark work *Persuasion and healing* (Frank and Frank 1991), the American psychiatrist Jerome Frank argues that comparable effectiveness arises because therapies largely function in the same way, in spite of their technical differences, meaning that they exert their positive effects through their shared characteristics rather than through the specific techniques that distinguish them. Boxes 5.1 and 5.2 present the proposed shared features and common functions of all psychotherapies, and even psychotherapy-like activities.

Box 5.1 Shared features

An emotionally charged, confiding relationship with a helping person.

A healing setting.

A rationale, conceptual scheme, or myth that provides a plausible explanation for the patient's symptoms and prescribes a ritual or procedure for resolving them.

A ritual or procedure that requires the active participation of both patient and therapist and that is believed by both to be the means of restoring the patient's health.

Data from Frank, J.D. and Frank J.B., Persuasion and Healing: a comparative study of psychotherapy, 3rd ed., Johns Hopkins University Press, Baltimore, 1991.

Box 5.2 Common functions

Combating the patient's sense of alienation and strengthening the therapeutic relationship.

Inspiring and maintaining the patient's expectation of help.

Providing new learning experiences.

Arousing emotions.

Enhancing the patient's sense of mastery of self-efficacy.

Providing opportunities for practice.

Data from Frank, J.D. and Frank J.B., Persuasion and healing: a comparative study of psychotherapy, 3rd ed., pp. 39–50, Johns Hopkins University Press, Baltimore, 1991.

5.3.2 **The Non-specific Therapeutic Factors**

The tension between the traditional medical notion of an active ingredient and the concept of multiple interacting general features is what drives current debate about the relative importance of specific types of psychotherapy. The issue in this debate is whether the techniques of a specific therapy are what are required to bring about positive change, or whether it is the non-specific factors that bring about change, where change is usually defined as reduction in symptoms. The active ingredient concept favours the former interpretation, yet to date there is no plausible explanation for the observation of comparable effectiveness of psychotherapy that is also consistent with the notion of an active ingredient, as this would mean that the theories from which these different therapies are derived are all correct.[2] Since some of them are contradictory, this cannot be possible.

There is no doubt that the mechanics of the various psychotherapies do differ in ways that might be quite meaningful to patients (like one of my patients who said of her former therapy experience: 'I was looking for something concrete, not someone who will sit silently'). Nevertheless, the active ingredient concept may not apply because the disease concept borrowed from the rest of medicine—that a mental disorder represents a deficit shared by all sufferers, which can be corrected using techniques that target this deficit—may also not apply.

Given the apparent similarities between taking a pill for hypertension and taking a pill for depression or anxiety, it might seem that the active ingredient concept is applicable to pharmaceutical treatments, even if not for

---

[2] There are certain important exceptions, such as the studies that demonstrate that psychodynamic psychotherapy is not particularly useful to diminish specific phobias.

psychotherapeutic ones. However, there are no known specific physiological deficits for psychiatric disorders; thus, it would seem that the medical concept of disease as specific deficit does not fit. Furthermore, while there are numerous somatic therapies for psychiatric problems (pharmaceuticals, electroconvulsive therapy, transcranial magnetic stimulation, etc.) their mechanisms of action are also unknown. In fact, individual pharmaceutical agents face a similar problem to individual psychotherapies. For example, we find similar rates of efficacy between different antidepressants (Clinical Evidence 2013a; Brooks 2012), and a parallel situation is found among the different antipsychotic agents (Clinical Evidence 2013b). Moncrieff has argued that psychiatric medications largely exert their positive effects in a non-specific way, producing a general drug-induced state that some people find helpful, rather than through precise actions on a precise disease process (2009: 14–25). So it seems difficult to support the claim that there is an active ingredient, when very different ingredients have similar rates of success while, at the same time, having unknown (or at least poorly characterized) sites and mechanisms of action. Again, the 'specific deficit-active ingredient' notion borrowed from the rest of medicine does not seem to apply.

What does all of this have to do with EBM? Recall that the purpose of the RCT is to isolate the effects of the putative active ingredient. I contend that, whether for psychotherapy or for somatic treatments, it is not clear that there is an active ingredient, in the sense that there is a specific feature to which therapeutic success can be attributed. This is not to say that these treatments do not or cannot work in the sense of helping people to feel better. Rather, I am arguing that conceptualizing these treatments as containing an active ingredient, and evaluating them as such, may unnecessarily limit our ability to understand how they do work and in what circumstances. It seems more plausible that there are several potentially active ingredients, that they might interact in varying ways and/or might not be easily separable, and that they might not all be operational in every circumstance. This type of situation calls for different research methods than the RCT, and it means that the evidence hierarchy may need to be set aside in favour of the best method given the phenomenon of interest and the research question about that phenomenon.

5.3.3 Placebos

Surely the fact that successful treatments (both medications and therapies) outperform placebos in RCTs justifies both the active ingredient thesis and the placement of the RCT at the top of the evidence hierarchy? A placebo is a substance administered to a control group in an RCT that is supposed to resemble the treatment being studied in every way, except that it lacks the active ingredient. Any greater effect of the actual drug compared with the placebo must be due to the active ingredient, and this is crucial knowledge to have when making treatment recommendations to patients who may accept the risk of side effects of a treatment if that treatment promises to reduce their suffering. The problem with this claim is that it assumes what is being argued. Prioritizing the RCT presupposes there is an active ingredient in the first place (because the RCT's goal is to isolate as much as possible the efficacy of the active ingredient). Taking again the case of psychotherapy research, superiority of a specific psychotherapy modality against a placebo is also consistent with the non-specific therapeutic factors thesis. It seems that any of the usual control group comparators, such psychiatric care or a general form of supportive contact, might simply be thought of as having a smaller quantity of these non-specific factors rather than being truly inert; therefore, a specific psychotherapy technique does better, not because of its active ingredient but because it offers a greater quantity of the non-specific factors. If we could establish a placebo control group who literally received nothing in the way of human contact and concern—say, recruitment and assignment to a waiting list by computer—we might have a comparator that lacks even the non-specific therapeutic factors. However, a positive result from an RCT of specific psychotherapy against a computer waiting list would simply tell us that something is better than nothing, rather than that an active ingredient outperformed a placebo. Thus, even RCT results showing the superiority of therapy versus placebo do not prove that active ingredients are necessary for therapeutic success. Positive differences between therapies and controls in RCTs are as consistent with both theses.

In reviewing research from a variety of medical specialties (e.g. gastroenterology, orthopedics, cardiology), Moerman has shown how the classic placebo from clinical trials (a sugar pill in pharmaceutical trials and a sham procedure in surgical trials) is far from being inert, having led to positive outcomes in substantial numbers of patients with a wide variety of medical conditions (2002: 9–66). Taking a treatment (placebo or otherwise) takes place in a relational context with certain hopes, expectations, and fear. Thus, he suggests that the placebo effect would be more aptly included as part of the phenomenon he calls the 'meaning effect' (2002: 14), in reference to the fact that the positive outcomes resulting from the use of placebos—since they are not brought about by an active ingredient—arise out of the culturally meaningful process of seeing a health care provider who believes in the treatment being offered, while believing that the provider has one's interests at heart.

The fact is, that large numbers of unwell, suffering people get better when they take sugar pills in psychiatric clinical trials. In clinical trials with positive results, active treatments are even more effective than placebos, but this does not negate the fact that the placebos were effective for some non-zero number of the participants. What is happening to these people and why? Clinging to the active ingredient concept focuses our attention upon the hows and whys of the active ingredients in the medications, and takes it away from the hows and whys of the mechanisms of placebos. EBM's prioritization of the RCT via the evidence hierarchy has the insidious effect of privileging the effect of the active ingredient while dismissing whatever clinically effective thing is happening to participants in placebo groups. According to the logic of the evidence hierarchy, the active ingredient should always be the more important focus of research attention. Is this the most appropriate focus of attention for psychiatry?

5.4 **Conclusions**

Evidence-based psychiatry has arisen from the direct application of EBM to psychiatry. However, I have argued that there are aspects of psychiatric disorders and their treatments that do not conform to the assumptions or requirements of EBM. As a result, the types of evidence permitted by EBM downplay the complexity of the experience of mental disorders, and potentially create a faulty picture of mental disorders. In turn, this evidence may not lead to accurate conclusions about psychiatric interventions. Evidence-based psychiatry may place psychiatrists in a situation whereby they believe they have knowledge about interventions they cannot justifiably claim to possess. If EBM does not improve our knowledge then it cannot claim to be an improvement over pre-EBM. This would undermine the imperative to practise, teach, and learn EBM. If, on the other hand, EBM were to revise itself to incorporate these considerations—by placing pragmatic trials or qualitative studies on an equal footing with randomized trials—the evidence hierarchy would be seriously compromised. In the absence of the hierarchy, we are back to gathering different sources of knowledge and judging various types of evidence on a case-by-case basis: the very situation EBM was designed to eliminate.

These problems in applying EBM to psychiatry would not be eliminated if EBM were abandoned. Indeed, the difficulties of achieving prognostic homogeneity and in quantifying outcomes are inherent to the RCT method, and therefore existed prior to EBM. Moreover, technical bias is part of any scientific method, as no method of investigation can capture all relevant knowledge about a phenomenon. EBM is certainly no worse in this regard than any other approach to medical knowledge. However, the lack of attention paid to these issues by advocates of evidence-based psychiatry suggests that these difficulties are inconsequential to our understanding of mental disorders. By failing to examine whether the demands of EBM fit well with the clinical dimensions of psychiatric disorders, evidence-based psychiatry promotes a particular view of mental disorders—namely, the 'specific deficit-active ingredient' concept borrowed from the rest of medicine. According to this view, mental disorders are understood exactly as other medical problems—conditions resulting from physiological derangements in the individual rather than because of psychosocial derangements, whether they reside in an individual, couple, family, group, or even the larger society. This change in orientation moves psychiatry away from its theoretically plural stance to one that is theoretically singular.

Rather than our understanding of mental disorders determining what counts and does not count as evidence, EBM's evidence is shaping our understanding of the nature of mental disorders and how we should intervene. This revision of psychiatry's subject matter has arrived on the coattails of EBM, and points to EBM's enormous influence: from shaping the conduct of research, to determining which interventions are deemed acceptable for consideration in clinical decision-making, and even to redefining the object of enquiry. EBM is not only changing our approach to researching mental disorders, it is changing psychiatry itself by influencing how we understand mental disorders, and thus the tasks of psychiatrists.

Psychiatry is also an ethical enterprise, whose basic ethical imperative—as in the rest of medicine—is to help, or at least to do no harm. To what extent does evidence-based psychiatry reflect and promote this or other values? The next chapter focuses on the ethics of EBM and of evidence-based psychiatry.

References

Akiskal, H. S. (2009), 'Mood disorders: clinical features', in: Sadock, B. J., Sadock, V. A., and Ruiz, P. (eds.) *Kaplan and Sadock's comprehensive textbook of psychiatry*, 9th edn. (Philadelphia: Lippincott, Williams and Wilkins), 1693–733.

American Psychiatric Association (2013), *Diagnostic and statistical manual of mental disorders*, 5th edn. (Arlington, VA: APA Press).

Bohart, A. C., O'Hara, M., and Leitner, L. M. (1998), 'Empirically violated treatments: disenfranchisement of humanistic and other psychotherapies', *Psychotherapy Research*, **8**: 141–57.

Brooks, J. (2012), 'Review: no substantial differences in efficacy or effectiveness between second-generation antidepressants for major depressive disorder', *Evidence-Based Mental Health*, **15**: 77.

Center for Drug Evaluation and Research (1988), *Guideline for the format and content of the clinical and statistical sections of an application* (Rockville, MA: CDER) <http://www.fda.gov/downloads/Drugs/GuidanceComplianceRegulatoryInformation/Guidances/UCM071665.pdf> accessed 3 April 2013.

Clinical Evidence (2013a), 'Depression in adults: drug and physical treatments' [website] <http://clinicalevidence.bmj.com/x/systematic-review/1003/overview.html> accessed 6 March 2014.

Clinical Evidence (2013b), 'Schizophrenia' [website] <http://clinicalevidence.bmj.com/x/systematic-review/1007/overview.html> accessed 6 March 2014.

Clinicaltrials.gov (2009), 'Sequenced treatment alternatives to relieve depression (STAR*D)' [website] <http://www.clinicaltrials.gov/ct/show/NCT00021528> accessed 5 June 2013.

Evidence-Based Mental Health (2012), 'Purpose and procedure', *Evidence Based Mental Health*, **15**: e2–e3 <http://ebmh.bmj.com/content/15/1/e2.extract> accessed 31 January 2014.

Faulkner, A. and Thomas, P. (2002), 'User-led research and evidence-based medicine', *British Journal of Psychiatry*, **180**: 1–3.

Fisher, S. and Greenberg, R. P. (1993), 'How sound is the double-blind design for evaluating psychotropic drugs?', *Journal of Nervous and Mental Disease*, **181**: 345–50.

Frank, J. D. and Frank, J. B. (1991), *Persuasion and healing: a comparative study of psychotherapy*, 3rd edn. (Baltimore: Johns Hopkins University Press).

Giacomini, M. and Cook, D. J. (2008), 'Qualitative research', in: Guyatt, G., Rennie, D., Meade, M., and Cook, D. (eds.), *Users' guides to the medical literature: a manual for evidence-based clinical practice*, 2nd edn. (Chicago: AMA Press), 341–60.

Goldenberg, M. J. (2006), 'On evidence and evidence-based medicine: lessons from the philosophy of science', *Social Sciences in Medicine*, **62**: 2621–32.

Gupta M. (2007), 'Does evidence-based medicine apply to psychiatry?', *Theoretical Medicine and Bioethics*, **28**: 103–20.

Health Canada (1995), 'The extent of population exposure to assess clinical safety for drugs intended for long-term treatment of non-life-threatening conditions: ICH topic E1' [website] <http://www.hc-sc.gc.ca/dhp-mps/prodpharma/applic-demande/guide-ld/ich/efficac/e1-eng.php> accessed 3 April 2013.

Healy, D. (2001), 'Evidence-biased psychiatry?', *Psychiatric Bulletin*, **25**: 290–1.

Holmes, J. (2000), 'Narrative in psychiatry and psychotherapy: the evidence?', *Journal of Medical Ethics*, **26**: 92–6.

Lam, R. W., Kennedy, S. H., Grigoriadis, S., McIntyre, R. S., Milev, R., Ramasubbu, R., Parikh, S. V., Patten, S. B., Ravindran, A. V. (2009), 'Canadian Network for Mood and Anxiety Treatments (CANMAT) clinical guidelines for the management of major depressive disorder in adults. III. Pharmacotherapy', *Journal of Affective Disorders*, **117**: S26–S43.

Maier, T. (2006), 'Evidence-based psychiatry: understanding the limitations of a method', *Journal of Evaluation in Clinical Practice*, **12**: 325–9.

McMahon, A. D. (2002), 'Study control, violators, inclusion criteria and defining explanatory and pragmatic trials', *Statistics in Medicine*, **21**: 1365–76.

Moerman, D. (2002), *Meaning, medicine and the 'placebo effect'* (Cambridge: Cambridge University Press).

Moncrieff, J. (2009), 'An alternative drug-centred model', in: *The myth of the chemical cure* (New York: Palgrave McMillan), 14–25.

Norcross, J. C., Beutler, L. E., and Levant, R. F. (2006), *Evidence-based practices in mental health: debate and dialogue on the fundamental questions* (Washington: American Psychological Association).

Oakley-Browne, M. A. (2001), 'EBM in practice: psychiatry', *Medical Journal of Australia*, **174**: 403–4.

Pérez-Iglesias, R., Martínez-García, O., Pardo-Garcia, G., Amado, J. A., Garcia-Unzueta, M. T., Tabares-Seisdedos, R., and Crespo-Facorro, B. (2014), 'Course of weight gain and metabolic abnormalities in first treated episode of psychosis: the first year is a critical period for development of cardiovascular risk factors', *International Journal of Neuropsychopharmacology*, **17**: 41–51.

Roland, M. and Torgerson, D. J. (1998), 'Understanding controlled trials: what are pragmatic trials?', *British Medical Journal*, **316**: 285–8.

Roth, A. and Fonagy, P (1996), *What works for whom? A critical review of psychotherapy research* (London: Guilford Press).

Schaffer, A., Levitt, A. J., Hershkop, S. K., Oh, P., MacDonald, C., and Lanctot, K. (2002), 'Utility scores of symptom profiles in major depression', *Psychiatry Research*, **110**: 189–97.

Seeman, M. V. (2001), 'Clinical trials in psychiatry: do results apply to practice?', *Canadian Journal of Psychiatry*, **46**: 352–5.

Straus, S. E., Richardson, W. S., Glasziou, P., and Haynes, R. B. (2011) (eds.), *Evidence-based medicine: how to practice and teach EBM*, 4th edn. (Edinburgh: Elsevier Churchill Livingstone.)

US Food and Drug Administration (2011), 'CDER: The consumer watchdog for safe and effective drugs' [website] <http://www.fda.gov/Drugs/ResourcesForYou/Consumers/ucm143462.htm> accessed 31 January 2014.

US Food and Drug Administration (2013), 'CFR – Code of Federal Regulations: Title 21' [website] <http://www.accessdata.fda.gov/scripts/cdrh/cfdocs/cfcfr/CFRSearch.cfm?fr=314.126&SearchTerm=duration%20of%20treatment> accessed 3 April 2013.

Wampold, B. E. (2013), 'The good, the bad, and the ugly: a 50-year perspective on the outcome problem, *Psychotherapy*, **50**: 16–24.

Wampold B. E., Mondin, G. W., Moody, M., Stich, F., Benson, K., and Ahn, H. (1997), 'A meta-analysis of outcome studies comparing bona fide psychotherapies: empirically, "all must have prizes"', *Psychological Bulletin*, **122**: 203–15.

Welsby, P. D. (1999), 'Reductionism in medicine: some thoughts on medical education from the clinical front line', *Journal of Evaluation in Clinical Practice*, **5**: 125–31.

Worrall, J. (2002), *What evidence in evidence-based medicine?*, ed. J. Reiss (Causality: metaphysics and methods, technical report 01/03; London: London School of Economics, Centre for Philosophy of Natural and Social Science) <http://www.lse.ac.uk/CPNSS/pdf/DP_withCover_Causality/CTR01-02-C.pdf> accessed 28 January 2014.

Chapter 6

The ethics of evidence-based medicine

6.1 **Introduction**

In the previous chapters I have described evidence-based medicine (EBM) and evidence-based psychiatry,[1] while at the same time discussing major issues in the debates surrounding how these concepts are applied in clinical practice. Where and how does ethics enter this picture? A hint that there is a link between EBM, evidence-based psychiatry, and ethics can be found in claims that ethical psychiatry ought to be evidence-based. Writing in the *Canadian Journal of Psychiatry* in 2000, Editor-in-chief Joel Paris asserted: 'Today, no therapeutic method will be fully accepted unless supported by randomized controlled trials [RCTs]. In other words, understanding disease and treating patients increasingly are dominated by an evidence-based approach.' Paris makes it clear that EBM is a required as the basis for legitimate therapeutic practices within psychiatry. He also suggests that it is not only the evaluation of efficacy of interventions that must employ EBM, but our understanding of mental disease itself (2000: 34). In 2003, Peter Szatmari, Professor of Child Psychiatry at McMaster University, wrote that '. . . the only ethical practice in [child] psychiatry is one that uses the principles of evidence-based medicine' (2003: 1). Here, even more strongly than Paris, Szatmari links EBM with ethics. In his article he views evidence-based practice in psychiatry as a more ethical approach to practice than what preceded it—namely, deriving treatment strategies from theories of normal psychological development.

The literature concerning ethics and EBM (see, for example, Kerridge et al. 1998; Miké 1999; Culpepper and Gilbert 1999; Leeder and Rychetnik 2001; Goodman 2003; Borry et al. 2006) considers various ways in which these two topics are related. Some authors imply that EBM itself is ethically neutral but has the potential to be manipulated for unethical purposes. For example,

---

[1] As discussed in the previous chapters, evidence-based psychiatry is merely EBM applied to psychiatric practice; I therefore use 'EBM' to represent the original movement as well as this disciplinary application.

Charlton worries that policy-makers might use EBM as a justification for denying insurance coverage for medical interventions that are not proven in EBM terms (1999: 257–8). Gerber and Lauterbach (2005) do not view EBM as value-neutral, but argue that the ethical critiques of EBM are not unique to it and are really critiques of medicine as a whole. Other authors suggest that the concept of EBM contains its own embedded normative structure, distinct from that of medicine, demonstrated by EBM's message that it is the only or best route to medical knowledge (Culpepper and Gilbert 1999: 830–1; Gupta 2003). Because practising based on the best knowledge is assumed to be the best way for doctors to help their patients, doctors who do not adhere to EBM may not be doing what is best for their patients and, therefore, may be practising unethically.

Chapter 6 explores the link between ethics and EBM, focusing on two questions: 1) Is EBM committed to certain ethical values? and 2) If so, what theory of ethics is reflected by these values? I address these questions, drawing upon *Evidence-based medicine* (Straus et al. 2011), *Users' guides* (Guyatt et al. 2008d), and the published literature on ethics and EBM as sources. The ethical commitments of EBM are not described directly in either *Evidence-based medicine* or *Users' guides*, but implicit references allow the reader to infer some answers. This discussion therefore offers a picture of the ethics of 'literal' EBM—that which appears in textbooks and published sources. I then turn to the major ethical issues that face the field of psychiatry and the way that the ethics of literal EBM does and does not help in resolving them.

6.2 Is EBM Committed to Certain Ethical Values?

EBM defines itself as the 'conscientious, explicit, and judicious use of current best evidence in making decisions about the care of individual patients'. In order to achieve this, EBM requires 'integration of individual clinical expertise and patient preferences with the best available external clinical evidence from systematic research and consideration of available resources' (Guyatt et al. 2008d: 783) (see Figure 6.1). This corresponds to step 4 of EBM practice, as discussed in Section 2.2.

How does the practitioner identify these three elements in order to be able to integrate them? Best available evidence, the first element, is determined by following steps 1–3 of EBM practice. The second element, clinical expertise, refers to the use of clinical skills (Straus et al. 2011: 1) that, presumably, are the result of medical training and practice. According to the authors of *Evidence-based medicine*, clinical expertise is what allows us to identify the third element, patients' values (Straus et al. 2011: 1). It is unclear what is involved in the

> **Evidence-based practice**
>
> is
>
> A. best evidence (steps 1–3) **integrated with**
>
> B. clinical expertise (which enables us to identify C) **integrated with**
>
> C. patients' values and circumstances.

Fig. 6.1 EBM's model of practice.

'consideration of available resources', as this does not correspond to any of the steps. Furthermore, when *Users' guides* goes on to define evidence-based practice, it mentions only that 'patient management decisions' are consistent with best evidence and the values and preferences of patients. Consideration of available resources is not mentioned.

EBM proponents acknowledge the importance of patients' values in clinical decision-making (Montori and Guyatt 2008: 1815; Guyatt et al. 2008a: 12–13), which is laudable although banal. The recognition that patients will prioritize their own values when they consent to, or refuse, recommended interventions is not novel. At the same time, EBM ignores the fact that parties other than patients might have values that are relevant to, or an unacknowledged part of, evidence-based practice. In the course of ordinary clinical decision-making there are at least two parties involved: patients and clinicians. Other parties might also be involved directly or indirectly: society, through the services or interventions that are covered through public insurance plans or the research it funds; private companies, through the services or interventions they are willing to cover or the research they fund; institutions, who might choose to develop certain programmes or clinics and not others; and family members, who might be involved in decision-making or expected to respond to the consequences of decisions made by patients. EBM is silent on whether, or how, these values operate within its practice.

While it is obvious that patients' values and circumstances can include ethical values, in what ways might they be integral to best evidence and clinical expertise, the two other elements required for evidence-based practice? Sections 6.2.1 and 6.2.2 discuss how ethical values may play a role in the determination of best evidence and the exercise of clinical expertise.

6.2.1 **Best Evidence**

Let us start with the question of whether values are at play in determining what is 'best evidence'. Clinicians determine whether a piece of research

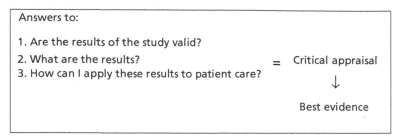

Fig. 6.2 The process leading from critical appraisal to best evidence.

can be considered best evidence by following step 3 of EBM, critically appraising the medical literature. The process of critical appraisal, regardless of the type of research study being considered, involves a structured approach to answering three set questions (Guyatt and Meade 2008: 6) (see Figure 6.2).

It is worth noting the kinds of questions that are not included as part of critical appraisal, such as: 1) Who chose the research question and why? 2) What version of health is valued by the methods used and the outcomes measured? 3) What interests are served by the interpretation of the results? and 4) Why does the journal want to publish this material at this time? These types of questions highlight the values that are part of the research process, that are embedded in knowledge claims about disease and treatment, and that are part of the consequences or implications of research. The answers to these questions reflect ethical values about the kinds of knowledge about suffering that are considered worthy of study, of dissemination, and of action in clinical practice. However, EBM's authors believe in a value-free view of determining best evidence, implied in the following observation: 'Linking treatment options with outcomes is largely a question of fact and a matter of science' (Guyatt et al. 2008b: 607).

6.2.1.1 Are the Results Valid?

In spite of the seeming value-neutrality of the actual three critical appraisal questions used for determining best evidence, they do invoke associated ethical questions. Consider the first question: 'Are the results valid?' Recall that determining a study's validity is to assess its 'closeness to the truth' (Straus et al. 2011: 3). In order to make this determination one must assess a study's design, because, according to EBM, certain designs are associated with greater validity. Evaluating study design includes assessing: 1) how the participants were identified and selected and whether they were fairly assigned to intervention or control; 2) whether the participants were treated the same throughout the study; and 3) whether the outcomes were measured objectively and whether the analysis was conducted properly (Straus et al. 2011: 63). In what ways might ethical values be relevant to determinations of validity?

The evidence hierarchy is effectively a hierarchy of internal validity (LaCaze 2009: 518–23). Internal validity is the extent to which a study has been able to measure what it intended to measure—in this case, the difference between the effect of a single active ingredient on a precisely defined outcome and the effect of an alternative (usually a placebo, sometimes an active treatment). In order to achieve a high degree of internal validity, researchers must conduct experiments under tightly controlled conditions. This will sacrifice external validity because in real practice conditions are different: there are often many confounding variables (e.g. multiple potential therapeutic situations and actions) and desired outcomes may be less precise or interactional (e.g. symptom reduction along with reduction in relationship conflict or work stress). Tight control is even more complicated in the experimental investigation of psychological treatments, where the nature of the active ingredient remains disputed and the number of confounding variables is potentially quite large. Adherence to EBM necessarily means prioritization of internal validity over any other criteria of good research.

Given the resources—money, time, personnel—involved in conducting RCTs, and the necessarily limited resources for research in general, it is ethically relevant to ask what the opportunity cost is of prioritizing internal validity. What types of research questions will not get addressed and what impact does the lack of availability of other types of research have on patient care? An RCT of an antidepressant medication may shed light on the rates and severity of certain symptoms and side effects for the duration of the trial. But when a patient asks 'how will I feel on this medication?' or 'why do people go off the medication?' internally valid data will have little to say, and potentially useful research that asks these types of questions will not have been done. This is not to say that internal validity is unimportant, but rather to recognize that privileging it over other types of validity is not a value-free decision. These values are ultimately ethical values in the sense that the types of questions that can be answered by the highly ranked methods may reflect the values of researchers about what it is important to know when it comes to taking medication, but not necessarily the values of patients who have to take them. What the patient wants to know may be directly related to what he thinks is important about how to live well.

6.2.1.2 What are the Results?

The second critical appraisal question is: 'What are the results?' This question is meant to direction the reader's attention to determining the size and precision of the effect of an intervention. Even though the size of an effect seems like a descriptive feature, it can contain implicit values. For example, the particular ratios or values used to express results can convey different meanings depending on their interpretation, and these interpretations can reflect value judgements. Some investigators criticize the use of ratios of relative risk because these might mask a very small change in absolute risk. A small change in the risk of death caused by an intervention from 0.01% to 0.005% will still be a relative risk reduction of 50%, although this might not be 'clinically meaningful' from the point of view of a physician or investigator. By contrast, a woman who is in remission from breast cancer, and who might have a relatively low risk of dying from a tumour in the unaffected breast, might wish to take any steps to reduce her risk of recurrence and opt for a preventive mastectomy, even if the absolute risk reduction is small. The meaning and importance of results require interpretation, and interpretation necessarily includes the interpreter's values, which are likely to differ between individuals.

Another example of hidden ethical values in research data concerns the threshold for statistical significance set by researchers. The threshold is the level beyond which the study's results were unlikely to have occurred through chance alone and are therefore probably attributable to a true difference between the experimental intervention and the comparator. The degree of statistical uncertainty one is willing to tolerate is a matter of values. For example, if one is trying to develop a treatment for a uniformly fatal condition with no current treatment, one might accept a lower degree of probability that positive results of effectiveness represent true effects. Offering some kind of treatment to patients who will otherwise succumb to their illness might guide the decision to allow greater uncertainty about effectiveness than is usually accepted. In other words, the greater the statistical uncertainty one will tolerate, the less desirable is the state of ill health one is trying to combat. Such was the case in the early stages of AZT (azidothymidine, an antiretroviral drug used in the treatment of HIV disease) trials, in which some AIDS activists pushed hard for AZT to be approved quickly, even with a great deal of uncertainty about its effects (both positive and negative), because of the universal and rapid fatality of AIDS at that time (Epstein 1996: 243).

6.2.1.3 How can I Apply these Results to Patient Care?

The third critical appraisal question—'How can I apply these results to patient care?'—most obviously involves the consideration of values. This step involves responding to four sub-questions (see also Figure 2.1 and Section 4.2.2):

1. Is our patient so different from those in the study that its results cannot apply?
2. Is the treatment feasible in our setting?
3. What are our patient's potential benefits and harms from the therapy?
4. What are our patient's values and expectations for both the outcome we are trying to prevent and the treatment we are offering?

The latter two sub-questions emphasize the importance of patients' values with respect to the outcomes of interventions. However, the second sub-question, concerning feasibility, implies values other than patients' values. EBM's authors interpret this question as referring to cost, availability, and implementability. Values—whether of institutions, society, or both—will play a role in whether to make available and to pay for certain interventions. If an intervention is supported by good evidence according to the first two critical appraisal questions, but no one will agree that it ought to be paid for or made locally available, then according to the logic of the third question, the intervention cannot be applied to patient care and this intervention is therefore automatically removed from consideration. This is another means by which values enter the critical appraisal process.

Molewijk and colleagues (2003) offer a concrete example of how the determination of best evidence must involve values. Their attempt to summarize clinical facts for presentation in a decision aid (about whether to undergo surgery for an abdominal aortic aneurysm) demonstrated that their choice of what facts to include, how to present them, and in what circumstances, reflected implicit normativity. They conclude that it is not possible to present a neutral version of the facts within a decision-making process. Instead, the facts themselves contain a normative dimension that not only informs the decision-making process but transforms it. In their words: 'The concept of implicit normativity challenges the traditional approach of bioethics [and informed consent] in which ethical reflection starts after the presentation of facts' (Molewijk et al. 2003: 70). Their observation is applicable to evidence-based practice, which portrays best evidence as a set of facts that can be considered in light of patients' values and preferences. *Evidence-based medicine*'s authors confirm this portrayal in their discussion of critically appraising clinical practice guidelines:

> So in deciding whether a valid guideline is applicable . . . we need to identify the 4 B's (burden, beliefs, bargain, barriers) that pertain to the guideline and decide whether they can be reconciled with its applications . . . Note that none of these B's has any effect on the validity of the evidence component of the guideline.
>
> (Straus et al. 2011: 131)

6.2.2 **Clinical Expertise**

What about the other element of evidence-based practice, clinical expertise? The nature of clinical expertise is a vast subject; however, for the purpose of this discussion we can note that clinical expertise involves the capacity to understand a clinical scenario in all of its complexity while considering and weighing the various factors at play. Expertise is also involved in weighing the options for action and making recommendations to patients about what intervention to follow. Since there is no formula for the exercise of clinical expertise the weighing process itself is subjective, in the sense that different clinicians will assign different weight to the various options of the decision under consideration and to the contextual features of the clinical situation. When it comes to clinical expertise about psychiatric diagnosis, some clinicians might weigh the appearance of certain symptoms more heavily than others. With respect to a particular treatment, some clinicians might weigh the possibility for symptomatic improvement more heavily than the side-effect burden, while other clinicians might take the opposite view. These types of weightings also reflect ethical values about which states of health are more desirable or lead to greater suffering than others. These values might be explicitly expressed in the course of decision-making, or might instead subtly play a role in clinicians' expertise by informing what they discuss with patient in the process of deciding about a clinical plan.

Ethical values inform all elements of evidence-based practice and are not only contributed by patients at the point of clinical decision-making. One reason that these values may not be so apparent in EBM texts is that they are obscured by the basic ethical platform upon which the very concept of EBM is based. The next section discusses this ethical basis.

6.3 **The Ethical Basis of EBM**

Why should we practice EBM? There is no evidence-based answer to this question. In other words, there is no evidence of the sort that is recognized by EBM that EBM is more likely to lead to a specific desired outcome, such as improved health, than pre-EBM practice (Norman 1999: 129–130; Shahar 2003: 134). Proponents of EBM acknowledge that generating this type of evidence is difficult because conducting RCTs of evidence-based practice would be methodologically challenging for the same reasons as studying any complex intervention. Furthermore, they worry that doing an RCT of evidence-based practice might be unethical itself, since it would require randomizing some patients to a control condition of pre- or non-EBM practice (Haynes 2002: 6).

The EBM texts point to specific examples of how, in recent years, well-designed RCTs have demonstrated that certain accepted treatments had done harm.[2] These examples are meant to illustrate that EBM is better equipped to tell clinicians which interventions work and which ones cause harm compared with pre-EBM. As a result, some authors have argued that failing to make use of EBM's scientific knowledge is unethical (Davidoff 1999: 82–3). But regardless of how compelling these individual case examples are, they cannot provide support for the general contention that EBM is the most effective means of achieving improved health outcomes. Instead, EBM contains an implicit mandate—that we should practise EBM. Thus, the basic conceptual structure of EBM is a normative one.

Where does this normative structure come from? EBM takes certain values for granted without making them explicit and explaining why they are good ones to hold. These values represent a moral starting point—the same one from which medicine as a whole proceeds (see Box 6.1). The first value is that we should pursue health. If not, there would be no need for EBM at all. The basic value in favour of the pursuit of health is a relatively uncontroversial one, particularly within the professional health care community. Obviously, the pursuit of health is the *raison d'être* of the health care professions; therefore, little time is spent questioning it. Controversies about the pursuit of health are more likely to focus on what constitutes health and how to achieve it. EBM is not a bystander in these debates given that its highly ranked research methods, and the techniques of critical appraisal, implicitly reinforce EBM's views of good and ill health. However, these issues are not discussed within EBM texts. Instead, EBM proceeds from the initial premise that if we should pursue

Box 6.1 Implicit values of EBM

We ought to pursue health.
If we ought to pursue health, then we ought to pursue the most effective means of achieving health.
Therefore, we ought to pursue the most effective means of achieving health.

---

[2] As mentioned in Chapter 3, EBM proponents frequently refer to two examples of RCTs that demonstrated that a treatment did more harm than good. These include the Cardiac Arrhythmia Suppression Trial (CAST) and the Women's Health Initiative Study of the effects of hormone replacement therapy (Straus et al. 2011: 69; Guyatt et al. 2008c: 70; Levine et al. 2008: 377).

health, then we should pursue the most effective means of achieving it. EBM concludes that we should pursue the most effective means of achieving health. These statements represent ethical values for physicians because their role is to help patients achieve health. Helping fosters a patient's capacity to flourish and live a good life, while harming thwarts this capacity.

By acknowledging patients' preferences in clinical decision-making, EBM acknowledges that there is variation among patients as to what constitutes health or, at least, what constitutes the desired outcome of interventions. This terrain is even more contested within psychiatry, where notions of healthy or normal mental experience are highly diverse. In an EBM context, 'health' is defined by the outcomes that researchers choose to investigate. For example, if the outcome for drug treatment of major depression is a 50% reduction in depression rating scale scores, as it tends to be in RCTs of antidepressants, then that is what 'good mental health' is.

In Chapter 3 I stated that EBM asserts itself through an epistemological claim—that EBM is the best means of securing knowledge about health; therefore, EBM rather than medicine as usual should be the pre-eminent method of pursuing health (see Box 6.2). In order to defend its assertion of being the best route to health, EBM makes two assumptions. First, EBM assumes that only if we pursue the truth (true conclusions about medical interventions) will we discover the most effective means of achieving health. This is a premise that most medical practitioners and researchers would accept as correct. They would point to the numerous successful medical interventions that have replaced previous unsuccessful interventions thanks to a more accurate understanding of human physiology and pathology. Second, and more controversially, EBM assumes that only if we pursue EBM do we maximize the likelihood of arriving at the truth (about the effectiveness of medical interventions). It is with these two assumptions that we are led to the conclusion that only if we pursue EBM do we arrive at the best means of achieving health. By framing EBM's version

---

Box 6.2 Implicit epistemological assumptions of EBM

Only if we pursue the truth do we arrive at the most effective means of achieving health.

Only if we pursue EBM do we maximize the likelihood of arriving at the truth.

Therefore, only if we pursue EBM do we arrive at the most effective means of achieving health.

Box 6.3 The (ethical) justification of EBM

We ought to pursue the most effective means of achieving health.
Only if we pursue EBM do we arrive at the most effective means of achieving health.
Therefore, we ought to pursue EBM.

of evidence as offering the most direct access to the truth about health care interventions, these assumptions obscure whatever values affect what counts as evidence in the first place.

The unstated value that we should pursue the most effective means of achieving health, and the epistemological assumption that EBM is the most effective means of achieving health, together lead to an inescapable conclusion: that we should practise EBM. This turns out to be an ethical obligation because if we do not practise EBM, we are not pursuing the most effective means of achieving health (see Box 6.3). This is a worse state of affairs for patients because it limits their capacity to live a good life. The implicit assumptions and values of EBM constitute an ethical justification for evidence-based practice—improved health through improved knowledge of the effectiveness of interventions, best achieved via EBM.

In Chapter 3 I discussed the debate concerning the role of ethical values within EBM. This debate focuses on challenging EBM's epistemological assumption—that EBM is the most effective means of achieving health—by showing that the knowledge upon which EBM is based is distorted in various ways. If the epistemological assumption fails, the ethical mandate to practise EBM is also undermined. Implicit in this debate is the idea that if EBM's epistemological assumption was correct, then the ethical obligation to practice EBM would stand. Is this true? What theory of ethics is reflected by this ethical obligation, and would we accept it as an appropriate ethical foundation for psychiatric practice even if we had no reasons to be concerned about EBM's epistemology?

6.4 What Theory of Ethics is Reflected in Evidence-based Practice?

EBM is committed to certain values—namely, the pursuit of health as defined by EBM—and is justified by an ethical argument rather than an empirical one. Yet the authoritative accounts of EBM do not explicitly identify or elaborate upon its ethical foundation, nor do they tie themselves explicitly to a particular theory of ethics. There is but one reference, late in *Users' guides*, in which the authors discuss the ethics of cost consideration in clinical decision-making:

> Some would argue—taking an extreme of what can be called a deontological approach to distributive justice—that the clinician's only responsibility should be to best meet the needs of the individual under her care. An alternate view—philosophically consequentialist or utilitarian—would contend that even in individual decision-making, the clinician should take a broader social view. In this broader view, the effect on others of allocating resources to a particular patient's care would bear on the decision , . . Our own belief is that while individual clinicians should attend primarily to the needs of the patients under their care, they should not neglect the resource implications of the advice they offer their patients. Neglect of resource issues in one patient, after all, may affect resource availability for other patients under their care.

(Drummond et al. 2008: 622)

Despite the ambivalence expressed in this passage, some authors have argued that EBM has consequentialist, rather than deontological, underpinnings (Kerridge et al. 1998). For an approach to count as consequentialist, it must at least accept that what makes an act morally right depends only on the actual consequences of that act (Blackburn 1996: 77). For consequentialists, what is morally right is not the character of the person who is acting (the agent), or the action performed by the agent, but the consequence of that agent's actual action. Utilitarianism, the best known version of consequentialism, has additional requirements.[3] First, utilitarianism is concerned with achieving a specific outcome: satisfying the principle of utility, which requires the pursuit of the greatest happiness for the greatest number. Furthermore, everyone's happiness counts equally in the evaluation of whether the greatest good has been achieved (Sinnott-Armstrong 2012).

6.4.1 Consequences

A consequentialist viewpoint must be able to specify and defend a consequence that is good in itself. For utilitarians, that good is happiness. For EBM, that good is improvement in the health outcomes measured in clinical research. The basic principle behind EBM is that interventions shown (using EBM-preferred research methods) to have a positive effect on participants in a clinical trial will lead, on average, to improved health outcomes for the larger population represented by the study group. Such interventions should then be preferentially

---

[3] There is debate about which criteria are necessary for a theory to count as utilitarian, but these are the minimum requirements (Sinnott-Armstrong 2012).

recommended to individual patients. This hints at consequentialist commitments. We ought to practise EBM because we assume it leads to improved health. And since improved health is what is considered to be good, we ought to practise EBM because it brings about that good.

EBM assumes that, generally, there will be concordance between what researchers consider to be improved health outcomes and the types of health states that patients prefer. Thus, if patients choose according to their preferences, this will lead to greater good in the form of improved health. But what if this assumption is not true and, on the whole, patients prefer outcomes other than those measured in clinical research or, at least, do not choose outcomes recommended by physicians?

At certain points in the authoritative texts EBM's authors make room for this possibility, emphasizing that the goal of clinical decision-making is to satisfy patients' preferences. For example, in discussing decision analysis, a method of integrating evidence with patients' values, *Evidence-based medicine* explicitly states that the objective of decision analysis is to satisfy patient preferences to the greatest extent possible. Interestingly, the authors even use the language of utility, where 'a utility is the measure of a person's preference for a health state'. In decision analysis, 'the "winning" strategy, and preferred course of action is the one that leads to the highest utility' (Straus et al. 2011: 115). Utility here is defined as a measure of an individual patient's preferences, but this does not seem to capture fully what is emphasized as good in EBM. If EBM satisfied patient preferences but led to no overall improvements in health, or to even worse health, this would seem to run against the imperative to learn and practise EBM. Furthermore, according to EBM, there are real limits on which interventions will be offered to patients in order to satisfy their preferences. Recall that assessing feasibility (cost and availability) is part of integration—step 4 of EBM—and will influence what intervention is recommended. Patients' preferences will be constrained by hospitals' or insurers' values about what improvements in health are desirable in light of costs, and what patient preferences they wish to satisfy (regardless of benefits to health). EBM aims to satisfy patients' preferences for certain health outcomes while acting within the limits that have already been laid down by the authority of the health system it is operating under. Thus, there do seem to be two distinct types of consequences that are good: improved health outcomes and satisfying (some) patients' preferences.

6.4.2 The Greatest Happiness for the Greatest Number

If we think of improvement in health outcomes and/or satisfaction of patients' preferences as being connected to happiness, we could view EBM as striving to achieve the greatest happiness among patients. EBM thus adopts one aspect of principle of utility, in that it focuses on maximizing happiness by maximizing particular health outcomes or preferences.

What about the greatest number? We can see how EBM concerns itself with this aspect of the principle of utility by the references within *Users' guides* to considerations of cost in the process of medical decision-making. For example: 'When making decisions for patient groups, clinicians need not only weigh the benefits and risks, but also consider whether these benefits will be worth the health care resources consumed' (Drummond et al. 2008: 621). Why does cost matter in EBM? One could imagine EBM existing without any consideration of cost at all. Cost consideration ends up playing a crucial ethical role in EBM, however. It enables EBM practitioners, in theory, to maximize the number of people who can benefit from (evidence-based) interventions. This moves EBM closer towards the goal of achieving the greatest happiness for the greatest number and closer towards utilitarian aims.

6.4.3 Impartiality

What about impartiality or equal consideration—the idea that everyone's happiness (health and/or preferences) matters just as much as anyone else's? Hints of impartiality are found in the population-based reasoning within the highest-ranked methods on the evidence hierarchy. The assumptions behind the selection of study participants, the types of data collected, the choices of analytic techniques used, and the types results reported are meant to provide information about groups of patients—namely, study samples and the larger populations they are meant to represent. These methods do not claim to provide information about any one patient but, rather, average results in a population. Within that population, there are people whose health improved, those whose health did not, and those who got worse. In step 4 of evidence-based practice, the practitioner applies research data to individual patients by making guesses about the extent to which the data apply to that individual based on shared pathophysiology with the study participants. In the case of bacterial pneumonia, where the infectious agent is known, this extrapolation may be relatively straightforward. In the case of mental disorder and psychiatric or psychological treatments this is considerably more difficult, given that pathophysiology is unknown and psychopathology remains pluralistic and contentious. But even if an individual patient is thought to be similar (pathophysiologically or psychopathologically) to a particular study population, the application of research data to that individual may not be of benefit because it will remain unknown whether the individual is more similar to the people in the study who got better, those who remained the same, or those who got worse as a result of the intervention. In this sense, EBM is impartial, not intentionally favouring or disfavouring the needs of any individual patient, but instead applying population-based data in the service of achieving the average improvement found in research studies.

6.5 **Beyond Consequences**

6.5.1 **Physicians' Values**

So far in this chapter, we have seen that in addition to patients' values, the other two elements of evidence-based practice (best evidence and clinical expertise) also involve ethical values. EBM does not acknowledge this. The authoritative texts of EBM describe its five steps in a linear fashion from the construction of a question, to a search of electronic databases, to a review of identified research papers according to the rules of critical appraisal, to clinical decision-making, to the evaluation of the whole procedure. The only values that are explicitly acknowledged are patients' values. The goal of evidence-based practice is to optimize health outcomes for as many patients as possible and/or to satisfy patients' preferences for the health states they value within the limits laid down by the health care system in which they participate. Improving health outcomes and satisfying patients' preferences are what count as good in clinical practice and are thus the goals for which clinicians should strive.

However, there is one additional aspect of ethical values that receives relatively brief treatment in *Users' guides* and that is the role of physicians' values in clinical decision-making. The authors note that EBM involves making clinical decisions and that a shared decision-making process is consistent with the principles of EBM (Montori et al. 2008: 648). There is some ambiguity in the text as to what the authors mean by shared decision-making. At one point they distinguish it from informed decision-making (in which the physician provides the information and the patient makes the decision independently) and 'clinician as perfect agent' decision-making (in which the physician makes the decision for the patient based on her knowledge of the patient's values) (Montori et al. 2008: 644–8). For the authors, shared decision-making involves both parties sharing information and values and coming to a decision together. At other times, the authors indicate that shared decision-making includes the first two types of decision-making as well (informed and perfect agent) (Montori et al. 2008: 648). In their influential framework describing the characteristics of shared decision-making from which EBM's authors draw, Charles and colleagues note that, at a minimum, shared decision-making requires: 1) at least two participants (doctor and patient); 2) that both parties take steps to participate in the process of treatment decision-making; 3) that information sharing is a prerequisite; and 4) that a treatment decision is made and both parties agree to the decision (1997: 685–8). Criterion 2 seems to exclude both the physician as perfect agent approach and the informed decision-making approach; in fact, Charles et al. claim that the three approaches are distinct rather than all being forms of shared decision-making.

For our purposes, it is interesting to note that the more restricted version of shared decision-making (the first version offered by *Users' guides*) includes the expression of physicians' values alongside patients' values in the course of clinical decision-making. It is unclear what role physicians' values play, or even what is meant by such values—i.e. do they mean the values of the individual physician or of the profession? Nor does the text specify what it actually means for patients and physicians to make decisions 'together'. What is the purpose of including physicians' values in decision-making? Is this consistent with EBM's utilitarian aims, in the sense that physicians' values should influence the calculation of improvement in health outcomes or satisfaction of patients' preferences? Or does their inclusion play some other ethical role such as fulfilling the physician's duty to tell the truth to the patient? These issues are not discussed. However, their inclusion suggests that there may be ethically significant aspects of clinical decisions, apart from the consequences of those decisions, that utilitarianism does not necessarily capture.

6.5.2 **Side Constraints**

EBM offers itself up as a complete model of clinical decision-making. This is evident in its evolution from its narrower origins in the critical appraisal of primary research papers (see for example, Department of Clinical Epidemiology and Biostatistics, McMaster University 1981) to its current status as an approach to guide clinical practice in matters of diagnosis, prognosis, therapy, and harm. Yet there are many elements of clinical decision-making and clinical practice that are not addressed by this model, such as personality conflicts with patients or families, genuine ethical dilemmas, the inability to reach consensus in decisions, etc. EBM has nothing specific to say about these matters, although presumably—consistent with its own logic—its proponents would champion the empirical study of techniques designed try to address such issues and the evaluation of these techniques in terms of their success in achieving resolution of the problems. In actual practice, such issues are addressed by drawing upon the guidance of larger frameworks of ethics and professionalism in medicine, institutional policies, regulatory authority policies, and legislation. These ethical resources have diverse theoretical origins, and therefore features other than consequences—such as rights, relationships, or physicians' duties—are considered morally relevant. For example, legislation concerning informed consent (which would be a backdrop to any evidence-based clinical decision about treatment) is not concerned with improved health outcomes or satisfying patients' preferences but with the duty of the physician to the patient, as well as the recognition of the principle of patient autonomy.

Where EBM stands on the importance of these other morally relevant considerations is an open question. Let's say that one could demonstrate in an RCT that informed consent actually worsened health outcomes for a given group of patients: it increased anxiety and decreased treatment responsiveness for a group of patients suffering from generalized anxiety disorder. It is unclear whether proponents of EBM would advocate abandoning informed consent in such cases or whether, regardless of the consequences, certain ethical practices operate as what the philosopher Robert Nozick (1974) called 'side constraints'. Side constraints are rules that forbid certain kinds of actions from entering into the utilitarian calculation of what maximizes utility. In this example, legislation requiring informed consent acts as a side constraint on utilitarianism, in the sense that whether or not to adhere to informed consent and the impact that would have on utility is a question that is simply not considered. EBM's authors have not explained how far they would extend the logic of EBM—i.e. whether and to what extent empirical data should trump ethical and/or legal considerations.

6.5.3 Virtues

Zarkovich and Upshur take the ethical theory of EBM in yet another direction. In their 2002 paper they focus on two key terms found in the original definition of EBM: 'conscientious' and 'judicious'—terms that have otherwise received little attention in the debate about EBM. The authors view these terms as referring to dispositions of the knower and, as such, they relate EBM to virtue theory. By this, they mean that the theoretical basis of EBM calls upon clinicians to mobilize and/or cultivate certain intellectual and moral dispositions. In their view, judiciousness is an intellectual virtue, while the conscientious use of evidence refers to a moral disposition.

> Indeed, conscience must be seen as connected to virtue theory, since the development of conscience is required for the development of a morally good person. Applying the notion of conscience to medicine, the EBM practitioner needs to make use of this virtue in order to be able to decide which of the current evidence is the current best evidence as well as to determine whether the best evidence results in the best care.
>
> (Zarkovich and Upshur 2002: 409)

Similarly, in examining the term 'critical' as featured in EBM's concept of critical appraisal, Upshur and I have noted that it captures two distinct notions (Gupta and Upshur 2013). First, it refers to certain cognitive skills that are needed in order to understand and apply the body of knowledge involved in the practice of medicine. Developing these skills is the explicit focus of the authoritative texts about EBM. However, there is a second meaning of critical that is hinted at in these texts. In the introductory pages of *Evidence-based medicine*, Brian Haynes attributes the origins of his commitment to EBM to an experience he had as a medical student.

> Brian Haynes started worrying about the relationship between evidence and clinical practice during this second year of medical school when a psychiatrist gave a lecture on Freud's theories. When asked, 'What's the evidence that Freud's theories were correct?', the psychiatrist admitted that there wasn't any good evidence, and that he didn't believe the theories, but he had been asked by the head of the department 'to give the talk'.
>
> (Straus et al., 2011: xiv)

Haynes does not seem to refer to the first meaning of 'critical' in the sense of the psychiatrist lacking the cognitive tools to make his own decision about the correctness of psychoanalytic theory (since he had already come to the conclusion that there was no good evidence for it). What is it exactly that the psychiatrist did not do in this example? He could have given a presentation critical of Freudian theory but he did not. Haynes implies that the psychiatrist lacked the courage to give what he believed was an honest assessment of Freud's thinking to the medical students or to his department head. This example reflects a second meaning of being critical—that is, to possess certain qualities such as the honesty and courage to question claims in the face of persuasion, authority, and social pressure. These qualities represent moral virtues. In other words, doing critical appraisal seems to require certain moral virtues in order to get the appraisal right. A commitment to EBM on the part of the practitioner is a commitment to the cultivation of certain virtues. If the justification for EBM is ethical, then part of this justification lies in virtue theory.

I have argued that EBM rests on an implied ethical justification and that the theoretical resources to support this justification lie in utilitarianism. However, there are certain elements that do not fit neatly into a utilitarian account of EBM, such as the inclusion of physicians' values in clinical decision-making and the possibility of accepting side constraints. It may be that EBM is based on a kind of restricted utilitarianism, accepting certain side constraints on its calculations of what maximizes utility, particularly those that lie outside the domain of medicine (such as legislation). At the same time, the terms 'conscientious' and 'critical' seem to refer to moral virtues—an ethical dimension of practice that also lies beyond the greatest good for the greatest number.

Despite this theoretical ambiguity, the central purpose of EBM practice, at least as it is characterized in its authoritative texts, is not to foster clinicians' virtues or to fulfil duties towards patients. This becomes clearer if we imagine that we could somehow establish that EBM did indeed foster virtue or fulfil duties, but did not maximize utility any further that what preceded it. In this case, there would not necessarily be the urgent imperative—as suggested by professional societies and accreditation bodies worldwide—to teach, learn, and practise it. Indeed, Djulbegovic, Guyatt,[4] and Ashcroft describe EBM as '. . . a practical approach to improving the quality of medical care by eliminating dangerous or ineffective treatments, promoting the use of well-tested treatments, and stimulating the evaluation of treatments where there is reasonable uncertainty about their merits' (2009: 159). In other words, we come back to the notion that improving health outcomes through the use of tested interventions is the main goal of EBM. The moral necessity of EBM is anchored in its supposed ability to maximize the good more effectively than any other form of practice.

6.6 Diagnosis and Treatment: The Central Ethical Controversies in Psychiatry

In the previous section I examined the ethical basis of EBM. To what extent does EBM's ethics converge with psychiatry's ethics? In other words, does practising EBM fit with the ethical aims of psychiatry or even improve the ethical basis of psychiatry, as some evidence-based psychiatry proponents assume that it would? Below, I explore some of the key themes that have arisen in psychiatric ethics in the contemporary era. I then discuss how practising evidence-based psychiatry does and does not address these issues.

The consideration of ethical issues has been an integral part of the development of psychiatry as a professional and scholarly discipline. While the details have changed as psychiatric practice has evolved, the main ethical questions have concerned and continue to concern the two primary tasks of psychiatrists: diagnosis and treatment. This stands in contrast with other areas of medicine, where giving diagnoses and providing treatment are themselves much less frequently the subject of ethical dispute.[5] Instead, ethical issues surrounding diagnosis

---

[4] Recall that Guyatt is one of four editors of *Users' guides* and a leading EBM developer.

[5] There are, of course, ethical disputes about diagnosis and treatment in all areas of medicine; however, the very idea of having a medical diagnosis or receiving treatment for that diagnosis is not controversial. By contrast, debate continues about whether the very notion of psychiatric diagnosis and treatment is ethical.

and treatment in other areas of medicine most often focus on access—whether receiving a medical diagnosis entitles one to treatment and/or social benefits, or not—whereas in psychiatry the very act of assigning a diagnosis or proposing a treatment may itself be considered ethically questionable.

6.6.1 Shared and Objective Standards

In order to determine who does or does not fall within their professional purview, psychiatrists must determine who has a psychiatric disorder. This task requires that psychiatrists possess shared and objective standards of what constitutes a psychiatric disorder. Psychiatrists have traditionally faced two major problems in meeting these criteria. First, to make a diagnosis, they rely primarily on patients' self-reports of symptoms. Because we cannot observe others' mental experiences, we can only make inferences about them. Clinicians have no independent method (such as lab tests) of verifying those statements, and instead are left having to assess their credibility and reasonableness. Unlike in other areas of medicine, specific anatomical lesions or physiological dysfunction have yet to be identified as the causes or even diagnostic correlates of individual psychiatric disorders. Apart from observing patients' behaviours, there are few objective methods of assessing most psychiatric disorders. Critics of psychiatry charge that the absence of objective verification increases the likelihood that psychiatric diagnoses contain value judgements—rather than scientific judgements—about what is normal and what is abnormal.

The second perennial problem in diagnostics is how to draw the line between normal and abnormal in domains such as thinking and feeling, which exist along a continuum and where the range of normal is very wide. Researchers can try to differentiate scientifically between normal and abnormal using prognosis (the development of morbidity over time). People who suffer from a true disorder ought to fare worse over time than people who do not. But apart from definitive outcomes (such as completed suicide), psychiatrists are faced with the problems of determining which outcomes should be considered morbid, and whether these outcomes were caused by a mental disorder, the innumerable variables embedded within people's social and economic contexts (poverty, abusive relationships, and unemployment to name just a few), or an irreducible combination of both. Thus, psychiatric diagnoses seem to be inevitably values-based, meaning that they involve pathologizing certain states of being as a function of normative criteria, such as difficulty functioning in society or subjective criteria such as the disvalue a person places on her experience of suffering. Comparing this to paradigmatic disease states in general medicine such as type 1 diabetes mellitus, the distinction is clear. Type 1 diabetes is based on objectively identifiable physiological dysfunction (absolute lack of insulin production by the pancreas). Whether or not the person feels well or does well socially has no bearing on receiving the diagnosis. In psychiatry, having a disease is based on whether or not one feels and functions well. Judgements about these questions reflect moral values about the kind of life a person ought to live and the kind of person she ought to be.

These nosological problems in the philosophy of psychiatry collided with the arrival of new drug treatments in the mid-twentieth century. Medications such as lithium and chlorpromazine seemed to reduce dramatically certain psychiatric symptoms, and these results strengthened the case that such symptoms had a biological basis like any other medical problem. Therefore, to diagnose and treat them as such was ethical. Nevertheless, the persistent absence of a system of objective verification of psychopathology, the limitations of the new drugs (both in terms of effectiveness and side effects), and the obvious failures of—and grave harms done by—other somatic psychiatric treatments such as malaria fever therapy, insulin coma therapy, and frontal lobotomies (Fennell 1996) kept alive ethical questions about psychiatric diagnosis and treatment through what came to be known as the antipsychiatry movement.

6.6.2 The Antipsychiatry Movement

Partly in response to these new drugs and their effects on patients, the antipsychiatry movement emerged in the late 1950s. Its leading exponents returned the debate about the ethics of psychiatric diagnosis and treatment back to square one by challenging the inferences drawn about mental disorders as a result of the new medications. They argued that psychiatric disorders were not real disorders at all, that mental illness was merely a label for describing violations of social norms, and that psychiatrists could not differentiate between patients with real and those with feigned mental disorders (Szasz 1974; Rosenhan 1973; Scheff 1984). These authors picked up on the basic conceptual and ethical problems of psychiatric diagnosis: if we can't be sure that psychiatric problems are real diseases, how can we be ethically justified in construing them as abnormal? Critics of psychiatry also highlighted ethical issues concerning treatment, particularly in psychiatric institutions. They worried that much of what we construe as mental illness was actually a response to the internal dynamics and organization of psychiatric institutions (Goffman 1961), and that psychiatric institutions and treatments—such as lobotomies and unmodified electroconvulsive therapy—were really expressions of social control rather than of therapeutic intervention (Scull 1977; 1979).

Certain feminist scholars added fuel to the fire by claiming that psychiatry was inherently misogynistic. Both Chesler (1972) and Showalter (1985) argued that, at various times in history, women have been considered more vulnerable to mental illness or more likely to be mentally ill by virtue of innate biological predispositions. As a consequence, they contended, women were more likely to be confined to psychiatric institutions. According to this interpretation, psychiatry was complicit in the systemic oppression of women. Popular observers also added their voices to the mix. Ken Kesey's 1962 book *One flew over the cuckoo's nest*, subsequently made into a film in 1975, became a well-known treatment of the same issues, portraying psychiatric diagnosis as a form of social control and treatment as harmful, even malignant (Kesey 1968). Both academic and popular critics had a profound influence on the public view of psychiatry, leaving the impression that psychiatric hospitalization and treatment were ethically questionable practices that often did more harm than good.

6.6.3 *DSM-III*

In 1980 there was a major revision, expansion, and dissemination of the *Diagnostic and statistical manual* (*DSM*) of psychiatric diagnosis, the dominant diagnostic reference text in North America (American Psychiatric Association 1980).[6] One of the goals associated with this third edition (*DSM-III*) was to render diagnoses more objective by making diagnostic criteria less open to psychiatrists' interpretation and therefore less subject to their value. *DSM-III*'s authors accomplished this by developing sets of criteria for each diagnostic category that were anchored primarily in behavioural signs, and attempting as much as possible to avoid diagnostic criteria that were theoretically derived judgements.[7] Roughly contemporaneously, the appearance of Prozac (fluoxetine) on the market in the mid-1980s heralded a new era of biological psychiatry (Shorter 1997); this was followed rapidly by several additions to the pharmacopoeia. Newer medications with more specific actions and seemingly fewer side effects than their older counterparts promoted a belief that psychiatrists were closer to an objective, neurological understanding of mental disorder. At the same time, a confluence of factors—including an evolving understanding of civil rights for mentally ill people and social policy that

---

[6] The *DSM* was first published by the American Psychiatric Association in 1952. Its purpose was to provide an inventory of mental disorders, along with their definitions, that could be clinically useful (American Psychiatric Association 1994).

[7] For example, in the first version of the manual, the disorders were identified as 'reactions', following the thinking of American psychiatrist Adolf Meyer, who believed that mental illnesses represented the reaction of a person to her life circumstances.

promoted less restrictive outpatient care—responded to some of the ethical concerns about hospitalization raised by the antipsychiatrists.

6.6.4 **New Activists**

A new generation of activists—psychiatric consumer-survivors, users, critical psychiatrists, and recovery movement adherents—has kept alive some of these conceptual and ethical issues. These movements are broad and include diverse viewpoints, including those that are cooperative with mainstream psychiatry and those that are critical of it. Nevertheless, they often share the belief that many of what are considered to be mental disorders are brought about and perpetuated, at least in part, by problematic social circumstances like poverty or rigid social norms such as those that define what constitutes appropriate childhood behaviour in classrooms. Therefore, mental disorders cannot be understood simply as objective, neurobiological processes. Some also contend that psychiatric treatments, even if scientifically based and/or concordant with patients' values, might do more harm than good (Everett 2000).

The metabolic side effects of the second generation of antipsychotic medications—which include significant weight gain, hyperglycemia, and elevation in cholesterol and triglycerides—are sometimes highlighted as an example that psychiatric treatments are still hazardous (Carey 2008). Some go further, saying that psychiatrists knowingly continue to downplay the negative effects of their treatments. As a result, these advocates question the ethics not only of psychiatric treatment but especially of involuntary treatment, which is legally permissible throughout North America and many other legal jurisdictions.

This summary does not provide a complete overview of all ethical issues relevant to psychiatry. For example, I have omitted consideration of how decisional incapacity can affect psychiatrists' work with mentally ill people. There are also major issues at the interface of psychiatry and the criminal justice system. This review does, however, capture some of the major themes from both historical and contemporary ethical debates about psychiatry. Ultimately, many day-to-day clinical ethical dilemmas in psychiatric practice result from these still unsettled debates concerning the legitimacy of psychiatric diagnoses, the risks versus benefits of psychiatric treatments, and the rights of psychiatric patients in view of psychiatrists' legal powers to detain and treat them involuntarily. Proponents of evidence-based psychiatry hope that grounding psychiatric diagnosis and treatment in scientific evidence will settle some of these disputes: at the least, evidence should establish the validity of psychiatric diagnostic categories, the efficacy of psychiatric treatments, and, therefore, the ethical legitimacy of psychiatry. EBM is certainly motivated by ethical commitments (see Sections 6.2–6.4); however, these might or might not provide a framework for addressing psychiatry's key ethical questions. Section 6.7 explores EBM's ethics and whether it addresses existing ethical issues within psychiatry.

6.7 Applying the Ethical Framework of EBM to Psychiatric Diagnosis and Treatment

EBM tackles the question of which treatments are effective, ineffective, or harmful at a population level. On the surface, it appears that the ethical commitments of EBM serve psychiatry quite well by identifying which of its treatments can improve mental health and reduce harm for the greatest number of patients. This could help the field to address the persistent ethical concerns that have been raised about psychiatric treatments—namely, that they do not help and often do active harm to patients. But this impression could be misleading. Could the values embedded within EBM work against its ethical aims?

The case of pharmacotherapy for adolescent depression illustrates the problem of how embedded values within EBM can undermine its role as a method of determining which psychiatric treatments work. The development in the 1980s of selective serotonin reuptake inhibitors (SSRIs) as a treatment for depression changed practitioners' attitudes towards initiating antidepressant treatment. Because of the belief that these medications had a more benign side-effect profile than earlier classes of antidepressants and were at least equally effective, physicians were more apt to prescribe them on a trial basis than previous antidepressants such as the tricyclics or the MAOIs (monoamine oxidase inhibitors), where side effects and potential lethality in overdose contributed to greater caution in their use. Extrapolating largely from studies of efficacy conducted in adults, practitioners also prescribed SSRIs to treat depression among adolescents. But in 2001 David Healy, a psychiatrist working in Wales, created a maelstrom in Canada when he publicly argued that SSRI use was linked to suicidality and completed suicide, particularly in young people. At the time, Healy was criticized as an irresponsible alarmist, and marginalized when his contract for a new position at the Centre for Addiction and Mental Health at the University of Toronto was rescinded by its Department of Psychiatry (Carey 2005; Healy 2002). Three years later, writing in the *Canadian Medical Association Journal*, Garland (2004) discussed the warnings that were ultimately issued in 2003 by several national regulators (including in Canada and the United States) about the potential for SSRI treatment to increase suicidality in children and adolescents. Pointing out the pernicious effect of publication bias, Garland argued that once the psychiatric community considered proprietary data (data in possession of the pharmaceutical companies that had funded the studies of SSRIs but were not in the public domain) alongside published data, it could conclude that—with the possible exception of fluoxetine—SSRI treatment in the adolescent population was ineffective and potentially harmful. Several authors have since addressed these questions of effectiveness and risk of suicidality in the adolescent depressed population (Cheung et al. 2005; Hall and Lucke 2006; Hetrick et al. 2007), and this debate has taken on a scholarly rather than a polemical tone.

Was EBM implicated in the reluctance to take seriously claims of harm caused by SSRIs? It seems quite possible that because claims of harm were initially brought forward on the basis of anecdote—a lower form of evidence—and were not supported by the publicly available RCT data, they were not given serious consideration. This example illustrates how EBM can lead us towards interventions that might be ineffective or even harmful. Technical bias keeps us suspicious of claims that are not justified on the basis of the highest form of evidence—RCT data. Source of funding bias and publication bias keeps the research literature—which is supposed to be our source of the most truthful information—focused on interventions that are commercially profitable, while giving private funders (such as pharmaceutical companies) power to determine which data are even released into the public domain. EBM's authors have expressed some concern about publication bias in *Users' guides*, and some efforts have been made towards reducing its impact (e.g. clinical trial registries). But at the same time commercially sponsored clinical trials continue to dominate the landscape of research in psychiatric therapeutics, and EBM continues to keep our attention focused on clinical trials. Thus, while EBM's utilitarian ethics appears to help psychiatry by attempting to determine which treatments improve health outcomes and which are useless or even cause harm, it might fail in these aims because of the embedded values that prevent accurate assessment of whether this good can be achieved. These values are common in the evidence base across specialties, but they generate greater ethical concern for psychiatric research because of the harm caused by interventions in the recent history of psychiatry. For critics, the case of SSRIs and their link to suicidality only strengthens the view that current psychiatric evidence continues a long tradition of psychiatrists claiming scientific justification even while potentially doing harm to patients.

If psychiatrists cannot be confident in the effectiveness claims of EBM-researched interventions, then adopting EBM might lead to recommending interventions that are not effective or bypassing interventions that are effective. Thus, EBM might lead to worse rather than better psychiatric care. Moreover, if psychiatrists know that their sources of information are potentially distorted in particular directions, adopting EBM—which does not take these distortions into consideration—undermines their claim of having more accurate knowledge than other mental health clinicians.

But even if we had access to all the clinical trial data, and even if we could be assured that source of funding bias was of no concern, there are still ethical issues at stake in psychiatric treatment. Whether particular forms of psychological and emotional suffering should be treated remains a contested area in psychiatry. Two examples are worth noting. First, in the debate about using propranolol to reduce the emotional content of traumatic memories to prevent post-traumatic stress disorder (see, for example, Henry et al. 2007), Bell (2007) notes that because it is not possible to predict who will actually develop the disorder after a traumatic event, offering propranolol to all patients who have experienced a traumatic event will pathologize a large percentage of normal emotional reactions to such events. Bell worries that this may medicalize a normal part of human experience. The elimination of the grief qualifier from the criteria for a major depressive episode in *DSM-5* offers a second example (American Psychiatric Association 2013: 161). The authors of this section of *DSM-5* have removed the criterion that the person must not be recently bereaved, which was previously present in *DSM-IV* (1994: 326–7). The worries here are similar to Bell's (Frances 2013: 186–8).

The ethical basis of EBM has a direct bearing on ethical questions related to the efficacy of psychiatric treatments. At the same time, it does not seem to engage with other major ethical debates in psychiatry—most importantly, the debate concerning the diagnostic validity. Instead, EBM takes for granted that psychiatric diagnoses are valid and focuses attention on which tools do a better or worse job of establishing diagnoses. In so doing, it avoids normative questions of whether certain experiences should be diagnosed as medical conditions or not. The philosopher Carl Elliott's article on apotemnophilia (2000) vividly illustrates the normativity of psychiatric diagnosis. Exploring the intense desire experienced by some to have one or more limbs amputated, he asks whether this constitutes a mental disorder, a fetish, a lifestyle preference, or some other phenomenon. Elliot describes the lengths to which some people have gone to obtain an amputation, including various forms of severe self-mutilation, because such people cannot obtain surgical amputations of their healthy limbs. I have used Elliot's article to discuss philosophical and ethical issues in psychiatric diagnosis with many groups of psychiatry residents and their reaction is always the same. They baulk at the idea that physicians should be involved in amputating healthy limbs, even with informed consent. And yet not all desires for irreversible changes to the body are considered to be abnormal. We do not tend to think of people who want larger breasts, differently shaped noses, or full body tattoos as disordered. We are prepared to allow people to obtain these bodily alterations. Why the difference with apotemnophiles? Ultimately, it rests in the fact that what they value about living a good life is so radically different from our own conception that we cannot believe it is psychologically normal.

Can EBM help to resolve these types of disagreements about the validity of diagnosis and help us to 'understand disease', as suggested in the quotation from Paris cited at the beginning of this chapter? An EBM approach to this issue might be as follows. We could design a tool that can reliably determine who is an apotemnophile and who is not. We could conduct an RCT in which some participants received amputation and some did not, and then attempt to measure their satisfaction or degree of suffering. Perhaps the results would be compelling: those who received the amputation might be very satisfied compared to those who did not. Yet these results would bypass an essential piece of moral work, which involves the determination of whether we want to identify apotemnophilia as a mental disorder or not. This judgement might be informed by scientific data, but it is ultimately normative in nature.

Even if we can agree that a certain condition—say, schizophrenia—is a mental disorder, there is more moral work to be done in figuring out how to treat it. Some might argue that the right thing to do is eliminate symptoms, while others might claim that a better approach is not to think of such problems in medical terms at all and instead to help patients learn how to live with the situation (Longden 2013: 36–9). How do we decide which outcome is preferred? Once a condition is considered to be a mental disorder clinical researchers tend to view the desired outcome as symptom reduction and, therefore, study the impact of interventions on the symptoms of that disorder. However, outcomes such as social integration, workforce participation, or standard of living may be more relevant measures to many people. EBM implies that following the evidence will lead to improved health and/or satisfaction of patients' preferences, without much consideration of what constitutes improved health in the first place and who ought to define it.

A final major theme in psychiatric ethics is the question of whether involuntary psychiatric treatment is legitimate. As long as we believe that EBM is a good method of determining diagnostic categories and treatment effectiveness, we might conclude that we have an ethical responsibility to see that it does get to the greatest number of patients to do the greatest good, even if through involuntary means. One must introduce ethical considerations lying outside the ethics of EBM, such as human rights, to determine whether involuntary treatment is ethical. This might be an example of how the utilitarian ethics of EBM, when applied to psychiatry, operates under side constraints.

6.8 **Conclusions**

In this chapter I have argued that psychiatry has struggled with intractable ethical issues relating to how we define mental disease, how we distinguish normal from abnormal, and what constitutes a humane response to mental suffering. Advocates of an evidence-based approach to psychiatry hope that the use of scientifically valid research data will address these ethically thorny issues (something along the lines of 'we are not imposing our values in diagnosis or treatment, we are just going by the evidence'). Yet EBM contains its own normative structure that favours maximizing good for the greatest number of patients. This might contribute to debates about the ethics of psychiatric treatment assuming we accept these as the appropriate ethical goals. As for questions of how to define mental disorder and distinguish normal from abnormal, EBM offers nothing explicit to these ethical debates. As a result, EBM cannot by itself provide the ethical substantiation for psychiatric diagnoses and treatments sought by advocates of evidence-based psychiatry.

So far in this book, I have examined the ethics of EBM and of evidence-based psychiatry as laid out in the key EBM texts (see Figure 6.3). However, the ethics

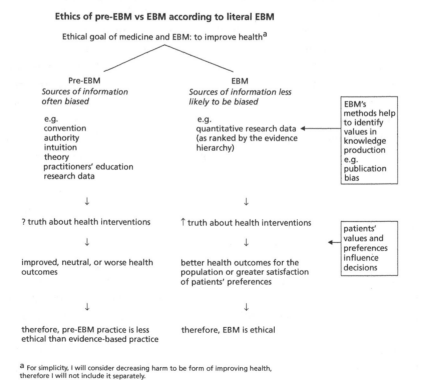

Ethics of pre-EBM vs EBM according to literal EBM

Ethical goal of medicine and EBM: to improve health[a]

Pre-EBM
Sources of information often biased

e.g.
convention
authority
intuition
theory
practitioners' education
research data

↓

? truth about health interventions

↓

improved, neutral, or worse health outcomes

↓

therefore, pre-EBM practice is less ethical than evidence-based practice

EBM
Sources of information less likely to be biased

e.g.
quantitative research data (as ranked by the evidence hierarchy)

↓

↑ truth about health interventions

↓

better health outcomes for the population or greater satisfaction of patients' preferences

↓

therefore, EBM is ethical

EBM's methods help to identify values in knowledge production
e.g.
publication bias

patients' values and preferences influence decisions

[a] For simplicity, I will consider decreasing harm to be form of improving health, therefore I will not include it separately.

Fig. 6.3 Ethics of EBM as implied by 'literal' EBM.

of evidence-based psychiatry lies not only in what is contained or implied by the authoritative texts that describe it but also in the views of those who are responsible for its ongoing development, implementation, and critique. Ultimately, EBM and evidence-based psychiatry are ideas that must be put into practice, and in that living context ethical commitments that are not evident from literal EBM might become apparent. In order to elucidate the ethics of EBM in practice, I turn back to the three groups of informants we met in Chapters 2 and 4: developers of EBM; mental health professionals involved in the development, implementation, and/or criticism of EBM; and scholars who have considered EBM from ethical or philosophical perspectives.

References

American Psychiatric Association (1980), *Diagnostic and statistical manual of mental disorders*, 3rd edn. [*DSM-III*] (Washington: APA Press).

American Psychiatric Association (1994), *Diagnostic and statistical manual of mental disorders*, 4th edn. [*DSM-IV*] (Washington: APA Press).

American Psychiatric Association (2013), *Diagnostic and statistical manual of mental disorders*, 5th edn. [*DSM-5*] (Arlington, VA: APA Press).

Blackburn, S. (1996), *Oxford dictionary of philosophy* (Oxford: Oxford University Press).

Bell, J. (2007), 'Preventing post-traumatic stress disorder or pathologizing bad memories?', *American Journal of Bioethics*, 7 (9): 29–30.

Borry, P., Schotsmans, P., and Dierickx, K. (2006), 'Evidence-based medicine and its role in ethical decision-making', *Journal of Evaluation in Clinical Practice*, 12 (3): 306–11.

Carey, B. (2005), 'A self-effacing scholar is psychiatry's gadfly', *New York Times*, 15 November.

Carey, B. (2008), 'Risks found for youths in new antipsychotics', *New York Times*, 15 September.

Charles, C., Gafni, A., and Whelan, T. (1997), 'Shared decision-making in the medical encounter: what does it mean? (or it takes at least two to tango)', *Social Sciences in Medicine*, 44 (5): 681–92.

Charlton, B. G. (1999), 'Clinical research methods for the new millennium', *Journal of Evaluation in Clinical Practice*, 5: 251–63.

Chesler, P. (1972), *Women and madness* (New York: Avon Books).

Cheung, A. H., Emslie, G. J., and Mayes, T. L. (2005), 'Review of the efficacy and safety of antidepressants in youth depression', *Journal of Child Psychology and Psychiatry, and Allied Disciplines*, 46: 735–54.

Culpepper, L. and Gilbert, T. T. (1999), 'Evidence and ethics', *The Lancet*, 353: 829–31.

Davidoff, F. (1999), 'In the teeth of the evidence: the curious case of evidence-based medicine', *Mount Sinai Journal of Medicine*, 66: 75–83.

Department of Clinical Epidemiology and Biostatistics, McMaster University (1981), 'How to read clinical journals: why to read them and how to start reading them critically', *Canadian Medical Association Journal*, 124: 556–8.

Djulbegovic, B., Guyatt, G. H., and Ashcroft, R. E. (2009), 'Epistemologic inquiries in evidence-based medicine', *Cancer Control*, **16**: 158–68.

Drummond, M., Goeree, R., Moayyedi, P., and Levine, M. (2008), 'Economic analysis', in: Guyatt, G., Rennie, D., Meade, M., and Cook, D. (eds.), *Users' guides to the medical literature: a manual for evidence-based clinical practice*, 2nd edn. (Chicago: AMA Press), 619–641.

Elliott, C. (2000), 'A new way to be mad', *The Atlantic*, 1 December <http://www.theatlantic.com/doc/200012/madness> accessed 7 July 2009.

Epstein, S. (1996), *Impure science: AIDS, activism and the politics of knowledge* (London: University of California Press).

Everett, B. (2000), 'What do consumers and survivors believe in?', in: *A fragile revolution: consumers and psychiatric survivors confront the power of the mental health system* (Waterloo, ON: Wilfred Laurier Press), 185–204.

Fennell, P. (1996), 'The age of experimentation: the board of control and treatment for mental disorder 1930–1959', in: *Treatment without consent: law, psychiatry, and the treatment of mentally disordered people since* 1845 (London: Routledge), 129–50.

Frances, A. (2013), *Saving normal: an insider's revolt against out-of-control psychiatric diagnosis, DSM-5, big pharma, and the medicalization of ordinary life* (New York: William Morrow).

Garland, J. (2004), 'Facing the evidence: antidepressant treatment in children and adolescents', *Canadian Medical Association Journal*, **170**: 489–91.

Gerber, A. and Lauterbach, K. W. (2005), 'Evidence-based medicine: why do opponents and proponents use the same arguments?', *Health Care Analysis*, **13**: 59–71.

Goffman, E. (1961), *Asylums: Essays of the social situation of mental patients and other inmates* (New York: Doubleday).

Goodman, K. W. (2003), 'Ethics and evidence', in: *Ethics and evidence-based medicine: fallibility and responsibility in clinical science* (Cambridge: Cambridge University Press), 129–140.

Gupta, M. (2003), 'A critical appraisal of evidence-based medicine: some ethical considerations', *Journal of Evaluation in Clinical Practice*, **9**: 111–21.

Gupta, M. and Upshur, R. E. G. (2012), 'Critical thinking in clinical medicine: what is it?', *Journal of Evaluation in Clinical Practice*, **18**: 938–44.

Guyatt, G. and Meade, M. (2008), 'How to use the medical literature—and this book—to improve your patient care', in: Guyatt, G., Rennie, D., Meade, M., and Cook, D. (eds.) (2008), *Users' guides to the medical literature: a manual for evidence-based clinical practice*, 2nd edn. (Chicago: AMA Press), 3–7.

Guyatt, G., Haynes, B., Jaeschke, R., Meade, M., Wilson, M., Montori, V., and Richardson, S. (2008a), 'The philosophy of evidence-based medicine', in: Guyatt, G., Rennie, D., Meade, M., and Cook, D. (eds.), *Users' guides to the medical literature: a manual for evidence-based clinical practice*, 2nd edn. (Chicago: AMA Press), 9–16.

Guyatt, G., Kameshwar, P., Schunemann, H., Jaeschke, R., and Cook, D. J. (2008b), 'How to use a patient management recommendation', in: Guyatt, G., Rennie, D., Meade, M., and Cook, D. (eds.), *Users' guides to the medical literature: a manual for evidence-based clinical practice*, 2nd edn. (Chicago: AMA Press), 597–618.

Guyatt, G., Straus, S., Meade, M., Kunz, R., Cook, D. J., Devereaux, P. J. and Ioannidis, J. (2008c), 'Therapy (randomized trials)', in: Guyatt, G., Rennie, D., Meade, M., and Cook, D. (eds.), *Users' guides to the medical literature: a manual for evidence-based clinical practice*, 2nd edn. (Chicago: AMA Press), 67–86.

Guyatt, G., Rennie, D., Meade, M., and Cook, D. (eds.) (2008d), *Users' guides to the medical literature: a manual for evidence-based clinical practice*, 2nd edn. (Chicago: AMA Press).

Hall, W.D. and Lucke, J. (2006), 'How have the selective serotonin reuptake inhibitors affected suicide mortality?', *Australian and New Zealand Journal of Psychiatry*, **40**: 941–50.

Haynes, R. B. (2002), 'What kind of evidence is it that evidence-based medicine advocates want health care providers and consumers to pay attention to?', *BMC Health Services Research*, **2** (3): 6 March <http://www.biomedcentral.com/1472-6963/2/3> accessed 27 January 2014.

Healy, D. I. (2002), 'Conflicting interests in Toronto: anatomy of a controversy at the interface of academia and industry', *Perspectives in Biology and Medicine*, **45**: 250–63.

Henry, M., Fishman, J., and Youngner, S. J. (2007), 'Propranolol and the prevention of post-traumatic stress disorder: is it wrong to erase the "sting" of bad memories?', *American Journal of Bioethics*, **7** (9): 12–20.

Hetrick, S. E., Merry, S. N., McKenzie, J., Sindahl, P., and Proctor, M. (2007), 'Selective serotonin reuptake inhibitors (SSRIs) for depressive disorders in children and adolescents', *Cochrane Database of Systematic Reviews*, **18** (3): CD004851.

Kerridge, I., Lowe, M., and Henry, D. (1998), 'Ethics and evidence-based medicine', *British Medical Journal*, **316**: 1151–3.

Kesey, K. (1968, first pub. 1962), *One flew over the cuckoo's nest: a novel* (New York: Viking Press).

LaCaze, A. (2009), 'Evidence-based medicine must be . . .', *Journal of Medicine and Philosophy*, **34**: 509–27.

Leeder, S. R. and Rychetnik, L. (2001), 'Ethics and evidence-based medicine', *Medical Journal of Australia*, **175**: 161–4.

Levine, M., Ioannidis, J., Haines, T., and Guyatt, G. (2008), 'Harm (observational studies)', in: Guyatt, G., Rennie, D., Meade, M., and Cook, D. (eds.), *Users' guides to the medical literature: a manual for evidence-based clinical practice*, 2nd edn. (Chicago: AMA Press), 363–81.

Longden, E. (2013), 'Listening to voices', *Scientific American Mind*, September–October, 36–9.

Miké V. (1999), 'Outcomes research and the quality of health care: the beacon of an ethics of evidence', *Evaluation and the Health Professions*, **22** (1): 3–32.

Molewijk, A. C., Stiggelbout, A. M., Otten, W., Dupuis, H. M., and Kievit, J. (2003), 'Implicit normativity in evidence-based medicine: a plea for integrated empirical ethics research', *Health Care Analysis*, **11**: 69–92.

Montori, V. M. and Guyatt, G. (2008), 'Progress in evidence-based medicine', *Journal of the American Medical Association*, **300**: 1814–16.

Montori, V. M., Devereaux, P. J., Straus, S., Haynes, B., and Guyatt, G. (2008), 'Decision-making and the patient', in: Guyatt, G., Rennie, D., Meade, M., and Cook, D.

(eds.), *Users' guides to the medical literature: a manual for evidence-based clinical practice*, 2nd edn. (Chicago: AMA Press), 643–61.

Norman, G. R. (1999), 'Examining the assumptions of evidence-based medicine', *Journal of Evaluation in Clinical Practice*, 5: 139–47.

Nozick, R. (1974), *Anarchy, state, and utopia* (New York: Basic Books).

Paris, J. (2000), 'Canadian psychiatry across five decades: from clinical inference to evidence-based practice', *Canadian Journal of Psychiatry*, **45**: 34–9.

Rosenhan, D. L. (1973), 'On being sane in insane places', *Science*, **179**: 250–8.

Scheff, T. J. (1984), *Being mentally ill* (Hawthorne, NY: Aldine; first pub. 1966).

Scull, A. (1977), *Decarceration: community treatment and the deviant: a radical view* (Englewood Cliffs, NJ: Prentice Hall).

Scull, A. (1979), *Museums of madness: the social organization of insanity in nineteenth-century England* (London: Penguin).

Shahar, E. (2003), 'On morality and logic in medical practice: commentary on "A critical appraisal of evidence-based medicine"', *Journal of Evaluation in Clinical Practice*, **9**: 133–5.

Shorter, E. (1997), 'The second biological psychiatry', in: *A history of psychiatry: from the era of the asylum to the age of Prozac* (New York: John Wiley), 239–287.

Showalter, E. (1985), *The female malady* (New York: Pantheon Books).

Sinnott-Armstrong, W. (2012), 'Consequentialism', *The Stanford Encyclopedia of Philosophy* (Winter 2012 edn.), ed. E. N. Zalta <http://plato.stanford.edu/archives/win2012/entries/consequentialism/> accessed 3 February 2014.

Straus, S. E., Richardson, W. S., Glasziou, P., and Haynes, R. B. (2011), *Evidence-based medicine: how to practice and teach EBM*, 4th edn. (Edinburgh: Churchill Livingstone Elsevier).

Szasz, T. S. (1974), *The myth of mental illness* (New York: Harper and Row; firs pub. 1960).

Szatmari, P. (2003), 'The art of evidence-based child psychiatry', *Evidence-Based Mental Health*, **6**: 1–3.

Zarkovich, E. and Upshur, R. E. G. (2002), 'The virtues of evidence', *Theoretical Medicine*, **23**: 403–12.

Chapter 7

Experts talk about ethics, evidence-based medicine, and psychiatry

In Chapter 7 I explore the various ways in which the three groups of interviewees (EBM developers, mental health experts, and philosophers, see Section 1.3 for details) understood the ethical commitments and implications of evidence-based medicine (EBM). Because ethics is a term of central importance in this investigation, it was essential to determine whether the interviewees had a shared meaning of ethics, and it turned out that they did. They consistently identified ethics in the health care environment in its normative form, whose purpose is to determine what is right and wrong, and why. Some participants also viewed ethics in relation to professional and legal standards.

Four key issues concerning ethics and EBM emerged from these interviews. The first issue focused on EBM as a manifestation of broader social and political trends. Those who argued for this idea believed that EBM must therefore reflect the values of those trends. The second issue concerned the question of whether EBM is value-free or value-laden. On this, participants were quite divided. Some believed EBM does not contribute a set of values beyond what already exists within the practice of medicine, while others disagreed and argued that EBM is motivated by its own distinct values. The third issue concerned the goals of EBM. If EBM has two goals—improved health outcomes and satisfying patients' preferences—which takes priority, and under what circumstances? The fourth issue concerned the question of whether it is ethical to use EBM as a tool for resource allocation. Again participants were divided, but this time along national lines rather than by discipline or by allegiance to EBM. I discuss these issues in more detail in Section 7.1.

In Section 7.2 I discuss participants' views about the relationship between ethics, EBM, and psychiatry. Drawing upon their perspectives enables me to develop an enriched model of the ethics of EBM. At the end of this chapter I compare the enriched model with the model implied by 'literal' EBM, as described in Chapter 6.

7.1 Key Issues Concerning Ethics and EBM

7.1.1 Issue 1: EBM is an Exemplar of Larger Ethical and Political Trends in Society

Mental health experts as well as the philosophers/bioethicists identified the political and economic context in which EBM has thrived as being central to understanding its values. These participants viewed EBM as emerging in the midst of broader social and political trends, including the emphasis on accountability and transparency in organizations, the prioritization of standardized processes in professional environments, the emphasis on risk management, the commodification of health care, and the political importance of social order. Participants did not claim that EBM was purposefully devised to reflect those values, but instead maintained that it could be understood as one of several trends or movements that exemplified those values.

> 2-1: '. . . the notion that we can automate the process [of providing mental health services] and mechanize it to the point where it's a kind of McDonald's production line, that, you know, everyone gets their dose of pharmacotherapy or CBT [cognitive behavioural therapy] or whatever the thing might be, and you know we know exactly how much it costs, and we know what it looks like and we know how long it takes to eat. I think these are kind of flawed notions and to some extent they tap into social and cultural pressures at a much higher level in mental health or even medicine.'

> 3-8: 'I think of evidence-based medicine as couched in all kinds of other movements out there. I mentioned the accountability movement already. So I think EBM arose as that sort of idea in health care: we need to reduce waste, we need to increase transparency. These are all democratic and cost-saving values. EBM came in as a great way to sort of facilitate those ends. So it creates a different ethical context where you need to justify democratically and transparently every move you have and the evidence provided by evidence-based medicine provides a way to do that. I don't think EBM changed that. I think it facilitated that kind of a shift in thinking that we needed to make everything transparent and accountable.'

The first quotation alludes to standardization and automation, values important in an industrial environment, while the second quotation hints at transparency and accountability as values in the political process, whether at the governmental level or in the administration of public services. One interviewee believed that EBM had been intentionally co-opted by politicians in order to garner control of medical practice.

> 3-1: 'The other people that were very interested in it [EBM] were essentially managers, health service managers, and politicians. And my interpretation of the reason why evidence-based medicine was picked up and pushed so hard in Britain was that it was a way of controlling medical practice. It had been very difficult for politicians and managers to control clinical practitioners because the clinicians were acknowledged to have the most important form of expertise. When evidence-based medicine

came in and asserted that the real expertise was actually an analysis of other people's research this put statisticians in control, but statisticians were funded and employed by the managers of the National Health Service and the politicians controlled the managers. It enabled politicians to control, at a very fine level of detail, the activities of clinicians.'

Likewise, some participants worried that EBM was a means of developing and maintaining an authoritarian relationship, not only between managers and doctors but also, inevitably, between doctors and patients.

7.1.1.1 Discussion of Issue 1

In their book, *The gold standard: the challenge of evidence-based medicine*, Stefan Timmermans and Marc Berg (2003) take up the question of the relationship between one of these larger trends—standardization—and EBM. In their view, EBM represents the latest of many attempts, dating as far back as the late nineteenth century, to standardize different aspects of health care delivery and practice. Rather than taking a position on whether standardization is something good or bad, they investigated how standards function in medical work and what impact they have. They examined a wide variety of standards, from chemotherapy protocols, to the use of EBM by residents in hospital rotations, to medical records. They concluded that standards play a dynamic role, transforming the relationships and the work in which they are used. Whether they are good or bad will be determined by their impact, context by context. This insight motivated them to write that '. . . the politics of standards should not be located solely in the regulatory-political environment from which standards emerge, but in the standards themselves. Standards are inherently political because their construction and application transform the practices in which they become embedded' (Timmermans and Berg 2003: 22). This notion offers an important perspective on the ethical analysis of EBM. Even if EBM can be understood as reflecting certain larger social trends, it is insufficient just to consider the values of these trends; it is also necessary to consider the ethics of EBM itself. Is EBM inherently ethical in the way that Timmermans and Berg see it as being inherently political? Or is it neutral, its ethics only evident in its implications? This question lies at the heart of the second issue—whether EBM is value-free or value-laden.

7.1.2 Issue 2: EBM is Value-Free versus Value-Laden

7.1.2.1 Value-Free

The notion that the ethical values of research funders influence EBM was a point raised by all three groups of experts. Some interviewees pointed out that these values do not belong to EBM and, in fact, that EBM can help to identify ethical issues relating to the generation and interpretation of research data, because the critical appraisal skills one needs to practise EBM are the same ones that help clinicians identify the biases in research and misinterpretations or poor interpretations of research data.

EBM developers did mention that patients' values belong within the EBM model, where they fit together with evidence and clinical expertise like pieces of a puzzle. This view is in line with the formal description of EBM, which states that EBM requires the integration of patients' values with research evidence and clinical expertise. Patients' values are one element among others that must be considered in evidence-based practice, but EBM developers did not think that EBM itself had its own values.

> 1-4: 'So [EBM is] a tool. It can be used for good or evil, et cetera.'

7.1.2.2 Physicians' Values

Some EBM developers noted that practitioners' values do play a role in EBM, particularly in clinical decision-making, but were uncertain as to how.

> I: 'I want to just go back and follow up on an example that you gave earlier, the multiple sclerosis example, and the physician who gives out evidence without thinking about whether the patient can actually afford it [an expensive, new treatment] and then puts the patient into a dilemma. Let's say that physician was aware that there was good evidence to support a treatment that was very expensive and was aware that the patient couldn't afford it, and furthermore, based on their relationship with the patient, was aware that sharing that information with them would put them into a dilemma. Is it evidence-based practice for that practitioner to say, 'I think I'm not going to tell . . . I'm aware of the evidence. I'm aware that it's a well-supported treatment but I think I'm not going to share that information because I don't want to stress this patient or this family or their financial resources beyond their capacity.'

> 1-4: 'It's clearly an ethical decision how you're going to present this to the patient. And I'm not saying how you should handle that particular decision. I'm saying the evidence can't handle it for you. It has to be incorporated into that process. For example, some of the considerations that might allow you to phrase it one way to one patient and another way to another patient include taking into account adverse effects or the difference between that new treatment that's very, very expensive and the next best treatment, which is pretty much as good, not quite, but doesn't have all the baggage of adverse effects or the uncertainty since we haven't seen the new one around for a while or long enough to know what its adverse effects are. So there's easy ways to maybe rationalize, in both the good and bad sense, of presenting different stories to different patients.'

A second passage further illustrates the hesitation of EBM developers regarding the role of physicians' values.

> 1-9: 'I don't know if the concept of EBM is defined by what information the physician offers up as an option. Is that still EBM? It's a hard question to answer, but that

would certainly be a situation where the physician would not be proposing one option in a discussion that is based on his or her values, so it could be seen as a narrowing or more of a circumscribed set of choices because of the suppression of one of them. So probably that would not be the fullest description of laying out all the options . . . EBM is definitely about values . . . [practitioners'] values are part of it. I mean it's naïve to think that they have nothing to do with it. But in that situation it would seem like the physician would be, obviously modifying or manipulating those things that are under consideration, presuming that there's some rationale for doing whatever is being suppressed. That's not the fullest discussion of all of the options.'

Others were certain that non-patient values should not play a role in EBM.

1-8: '. . . my particular position is the physicians' values and the researchers' values are irrelevant. Completely, utterly, and totally irrelevant. Now, within the shared decision-making frameworks, which my understanding may still be a little superficial on those, but as I understand it, the physician puts their values and preferences on the table, the patient puts theirs, and somehow they work things out. I'm not sure what the physician's values and preferences, why they should have any bearing on this matter personally.'

Mental health experts and philosophers/bioethicists took a different perspective. To them, values form the entire framework of medical practice.

2-1: '. . . what is the purpose of mental health care? Why are we there? What are we actually trying to achieve? And what's the relative balance between what we think is in the person's best interest and what they think is in their best interest? These kind of discussions just don't have invariant solutions, they're not amenable to automated problem-solving, they're not sensible things to try and address through manualized means, they're values. . .'

7.1.2.3 Hidden Values

Philosophy and bioethics experts pointed out that EBM itself could contain hidden values, noting that a limited focus on patients' values could divert attention away from other ethical values operating as part of the framework. For example, some worried that EBM contained its own conflicts of interest. The generation of randomized controlled trial (RCT) data, an essential component of EBM, often involves relationships between investigators and private industry. These relationships could then introduce biases into researchers' work. Thus, in order to pursue a career devoted to producing high-quality evidence, one might have to pursue relationships that work against the disinterested stance championed by EBM.

Some of the philosophy experts went further, arguing that EBM does not acknowledge its embedded values, and that EBM proponents were simply wrong to believe that individual practitioners can be neutral in their application of the model. Thus, by itself, EBM cannot identify and be critical of values within its own model, or even in those external to EBM that influence it.

> 3-8: 'My criticism is that they [EBM's authors] claim to be value-neutral and many of their methods attest to that. For example, that idea of the critical appraiser, that somehow if they have the right methods and they know how to use them, that they're somehow going to be able to get past all that. It's just not true. Not to say that all judgments are the same. There are better clinical judgments than others, but it's not about who has values and who doesn't. It's about which values are playing in.'

Finally, one participant believed that EBM's attempt to handle patients' values, through techniques such as decision analysis, actually glosses over values by trying to concretize them, and does not do justice to the true complexity of how people evaluate various health states.

> 3-10: 'I mean, the whole idea of patient utilities I find kind of laughable. The idea that you can take a patient's goals and values and quantify them in some sort of way or label them and say, 'Oh well, you're a risk-averse patient, okay? . . . based on how you filled out this questionnaire, you're a risk-averse patient, and so risk-averse patients shouldn't get this chemotherapeutic regimen and should instead go to palliative care'. And the patient says: 'Well you know what? I want the chemotherapy.' So far, when evidence-based medicine attempts to measure, quantify, and incorporate goals, values, patient preferences in a more objective way, I think it is problematic and not ideal.'

7.1.2.4 Discussion of Issue 2

Some participants suggested that the basic questions of clinical practice are questions about values rather than questions about medical facts. Therefore, values are not merely one element in clinical decision-making, but are the foundation upon which practice rests. Clinical practice, whether evidence-based or otherwise, has to be based on these values.

Where do these values come from? Are they part of EBM or do they come from somewhere else? Some experts believed that the values of medicine were well established and provided a moral framework for the clinical practice. EBM is obliged to operate within this framework. In other words, in practice, EBM takes on the values of medicine in general. Gerber and Lauterbach (2005) discuss this question in some detail. For them, EBM is not value-free, but the values of EBM are just the values of medicine. They identify several issues which they believe are criticisms of EBM on ethical grounds, but they could equally be criticisms of medicine. These include:

1. Claim of truth
2. Claim of objectivity
3. Intrinsic normativity
4. Source of funding bias
5. Hierarchy of knowledge
6. Lack of social awareness

7. Publication bias

8. Population-centered versus individuum-centered

(Gerber and Lauterbach 2005: 63)

The authors are correct in identifying certain values in common between EBM and medicine, in the sense that any current biomedical approach takes as central the ethical mission to improve health, with the accompanying belief that this will be best achieved by scientific (truthful) accounts of disease and treatment. Furthermore, any approach to medicine will be subject to the values of the society and institutions in which it exists (e.g. medical research was subject to source of funding bias even before EBM). Nevertheless, EBM's authors claimed it to be a 'new paradigm' (Evidence-Based Medicine Working Group 1992: 2420), contrasting it with pre-EBM medicine in its basic assumptions. One of these assumptions is that by focusing on the research methods highly ranked by the evidence hierarchy, EBM offers privileged access to medical knowledge in the domains of diagnosis, prognosis, treatment, and harm, compared with other approaches to medicine. Having made this move, the authors go on to defend EBM on ethical grounds—we ought to practice EBM because it is more likely to lead to improved health compared to pre-EBM medicine. Our concepts of health and disease are normative; therefore, when EBM claims superiority in improving health, it is making an epistemological claim about its methods, as well as an ethical claim about what counts as health. In short, the kinds of ethical issues that crop up for EBM are similar to those in medicine, but the way that EBM responds to these issues is different.

Mental health interviewees expressed the worry that EBM was being used to determine which treatment options clinicians can offer to patients, and that the options it permits do not constitute a value-neutral list but instead are shaped by the values of EBM, in particular privileging those options that could be studied most easily using the methods of EBM. Participants from the United Kingdom offered the example of nationally mandated treatment pathways in their country, through which the values of EBM constrain patient choice of treatment options. By contrast, others believed that the values of EBM work in favour of patients. By subjecting interventions to empirical investigation, EBM was potentially giving practitioners greater knowledge about their efficacy, which ultimately improved patient care. Moreover, by offering this knowledge, EBM can strengthen the informed consent process by enabling the practitioner to discuss the evidence behind the various treatment options, mentioning when evidence was lacking or of poor quality, or when it disfavoured an available intervention.[1] This too was viewed as an improvement to patient care thanks to EBM.

---

[1] For further discussion on this point, see the papers by Hope (2002) and Parker (2001).

If we compare the interviewee groups along the issue of whether EBM is value-free or value-laden, an important pattern emerges. EBM developers describe EBM as a value-neutral tool that evolved through developments in medical research. They are ambivalent about acknowledging the role of values in the model, including practitioners' values, even though these are explicitly mentioned as part of shared decision-making and considered to be part of evidence-based practice. Even patients' values are portrayed objectively, meaning that: 1) they are viewed from the point of view of the practitioner, who can then observe and describe them neutrally as 'patient A's values'; 2) they can be thought of as a type of information alongside research data that must be taken into consideration; and 3) they can be quantified and mathematical operations can then be performed upon them.

Mental health experts were inclined to see the ways in which all of clinical practice is imbued by ethical values. Nevertheless, there was a divide among mental health experts. Some agreed with EBM developers that as a concept EBM was value-free, even if it manifested certain values when put into practice. Others agreed with the broader view expressed by the philosophers that ethical values are part of EBM, just as they are part of all human endeavours. While only three of the 33 interviewees spontaneously described EBM as utilitarian in such terms, many more participants recognized that EBM is orientated towards maximizing good for the greatest number. However, they noted that the ethics of medical practice requires consideration of individual good, and that sometimes the good of the many must be sacrificed for the good of one.

7.1.3 Issue 3: Improved Health Outcomes versus Satisfying Patients' Preferences: Which takes Priority?

EBM seems to have two goals (see Chapter 6): one is to improve health outcomes and the other is to satisfy patients' preferences. What happens when these two goals conflict; for example, if an intervention will improve health outcomes but not satisfy patients' preferences or an intervention will not improve health outcomes but will satisfy patients' preferences? In theory, the first alternative is easy to answer. If a proposed intervention does not satisfy a patient's preference, he will refuse to accept it. The difficulty begins at that point. What should the practitioner propose next? To what extent can an intervention be ineffective, yet still be ethically acceptable under EBM because it will satisfy patients' preferences?

One participant offers a hint that helps in answering this question.

> 1-1: 'I think when we know something doesn't work, or when we know it causes harm, or when we know that something doesn't work as well as an alternative, to continue to cling to it, to continue to treat patients with it is a failure of ethics . . .'

7.1.3.1 Discussion of Issue 3

In supporting EBM, some participants made reference to past failed or harmful treatments. The Cardiac Arrhythmia Suppression Trial (CAST) was a frequently referenced example (see Section 3.2). This trial established that certain drugs prescribed to decrease the rates of fatal arrhythmias in the post-myocardial infarction period actually increased their frequency and contributed to excess mortality (ClinicalTrials.gov 2005). In this example, the harm lay in the intervention doing the very opposite of what it was thought to do. Inasmuch as adhering to EBM enables practitioners to avoid offering harmful interventions such as these drugs, it works towards improving health outcomes. Under these circumstances, the goal of improved health outcomes trumps the goal of satisfying patients' preferences in that, even if a patient requested an intervention known to be harmful, it would be ethical—perhaps even obligatory, as this participant suggests—for the practitioner to refuse to offer it.

The CAST example stands out, however, because it is exceptional in identifying a definitive harm. By contrast, the vast majority of clinical trials in psychiatry are designed to investigate whether there is a difference in effect between a placebo and an active drug. In other words, these trials are seeking to investigate relative effectiveness (on a target condition) and relative harms (side effects). The comment from interviewee 1-1 (see the quotation in 7.1.3) highlights this fact—that we learn different kinds of things about interventions from clinical research. In addition to the kind of definitive harm illustrated by the CAST example (doing the opposite of what we thought), worse health can result when an intervention does not work (it is equally effective to placebo), when it is less effective than an existing treatment, or, to add to participant 1-1's comment, when it works as well or better than an alternative but causes greater side effects.

Most clinical trials do not demonstrate a definitive harm in which concern for health outcomes trumps patients' preferences and the intervention is removed from the menu of options. Instead, the results of clinical research usually contribute to clinical discussions about the trade-off between effectiveness and side effects. In treatment decision-making, for example, clinicians and patients have to decide whether the chances of the treatment working are worth the risk of developing side effects (including weighing the gravity of those side effects). In these cases, the ethical goal of EBM is to satisfy patients' preferences, meaning to select the intervention that corresponds with patients' trade-offs between potential benefits and harms. In theory, all treatments that are not definitively harmful should be on the menu of available treatment options, and the ethical questions concern whose ethical values play a role in determining what kinds of positive effects are to be valued, what kinds of harm are to be avoided, and how this information is framed and presented.

However, the following exchange between participant 2-9 and me suggests that definitive harm is not the only reason that certain interventions do not make it onto the menu of available options.

> I: 'What if somebody wants something that's not evidence-based? What do you do about that situation?'
>
> 2-9: As a doctor I'd say, "Well, there's no evidence for that. It's up to you".
>
> I: 'So if they say, "No, I really do want that thing".'
>
> 2-9: 'Oh I see . . . say, "I really want some . . . benzodiazepines". I would say, "No, I can't do that because I'm very sure that it is a bad idea to give you long-term benzodiazepines. So I feel that would be against my ethical principle directing your interests".'

Although these types of situations are cast as ones in which evidence trumps patient preferences because of the potential for harm, the evidence of harm in these cases is determined in part by the practitioner's values about what kinds of outcomes are appropriate or not. The benzodiazepine example is germane to psychiatry. Many patients use benzodiazepines to help them fall or stay asleep. And while practitioners can marshal many good health-related reasons why this is not the best way of facilitating healthy sleep patterns in patients with insomnia, some patients will prefer to take benzodiazepines, including on a long-term basis, risking the harms that practitioners fear. When a practitioner refuses to prescribe this way, she does so in accordance with her own values about what a good health outcome is. Calling this evidence obscures the practitioner's ethical values behind this clinical decision to withhold prescription.

The passage discussed here suggests that physicians' values do play a role in determining treatment options, even if they do not recognize it. If a patient wants something that a clinician decides is unsuitable based on her interpretation of research data, this participant believed that it is consistent with EBM to exclude that option from the menu. Thus, even in the absence of definitive harms, patients' preferences do not necessarily prevail. Other parties' values weigh in. EBM texts recognize that the menu of treatment options is shaped by what is locally available and what the insurer or patient will pay for. But recall that EBM developers (see Section 7.1.2.2) were uncertain to what extent practitioners' values should also influence which treatment options are offered. Thus, determining how to weigh improved health outcomes against patients' preferences, and the role of physicians' values in that process in particular, remains unsettled.

7.1.4 **Issue 4: Should EBM be Used for Resource Allocation?**

The final issue raised by the interviewees concerned EBM's role vis-à-vis resource allocation. There were divergences on this topic among the participants, but in this case, instead of being based on disciplinary background, convergences and divergences fell quite strikingly along national lines, regardless of whether the participant was a proponent or critic of EBM.

7.1.4.1 Discussion of Issue 4

Some experts believed that EBM had a significant role to play in the just allocation of resources, others were ambivalent about this use of EBM, and still others believed that it was exactly this aspect of EBM that made it unethical. Participants from the United Kingdom, where EBM has been adopted explicitly by the National Institute for Health and Care Excellence (NICE) as a tool in health resource allocation, were deeply concerned about the extent to which this approach has led to the disregard of individual patient values and needs. A related concern was the extent to which the use of EBM for resource allocation forced practitioners to act unethically, by setting aside their knowledge of individual patients or local circumstances and providing treatments that were inappropriate in specific circumstances.

Participants in Canada, while recognizing that resource allocation was a central part of health policy-making, were ambivalent about what role EBM should play in this task. In an early defence of EBM, Sackett (who spent most of his career in Canada) and colleagues claimed that it was a misuse of EBM to treat it as a cost-cutting tool. Instead, they wrote: 'Doctors practicing evidence-based medicine will identify and apply the most efficacious interventions to maximize the quality and quantity of life for individual patients; this may raise rather than lower the cost of their care' (1996: 72). On the other hand, *Users' guides* now directly considers consideration of cost to be part of evidence-based practice (2008: 783). It is therefore understandable that even the EBM developers I interviewed were uncertain on this point.

Participants from the United States, where EBM is used by private insurance companies to determine eligible or ineligible treatments, were divided about whether this was an ethical use of EBM or not. On the one hand there was a similar worry to that expressed by UK participants that such determinations offered worse care, by applying population-derived data to all holders of a given policy without taking into account individual variation or needs. On the other hand some pointed out that EBM allowed treatment eligibility to be determined on rational grounds. The divergence between the United Kingdom and

United States on this point seemed to relate to the results of resource allocation. In the United Kingdom the use of EBM seemed to narrow practitioners' and patients' options, while in the United States, at least in some situations, it may have led to a fairer allocation of services than what had occurred previously.

Participant 3-5 speculated as to why some people may be ambivalent about the role EBM has to play in resource allocation. Asked whether EBM includes a commitment to resource allocation, this expert gave the following answer.

> 3-5: 'I think it is part of it and you can't really talk about evidence-based medicine without talking about it, if for no other reason than historical ones that the founding text of the movement is Archie Cochrane's *Effectiveness and efficiency*, where effectiveness and efficiency are linked together in the title but also in the analysis throughout the book. And it places the need to use resources efficiently at the heart of what it is to organize a just and effective health service. That said, one of the reasons why supporters of evidence-based medicine sometimes avoid engaging in debates about cost–effectiveness is because the vast majority of treatments have never been tested, so they say . . . so simply to say, "Well we can't allocate resources except on the basis of robust clinical evidence" would be to say "Well we're not going to do 95% of medicine at all".'

7.2 The Relationship between Ethical Practice and Evidence-based Practice

Experts from all three of the interview groups, proponents and critics alike, stated—or alluded to—the idea that evidence-based practice is rational, and rational practice is ethically good. Western medicine takes as fundamental the idea that a scientific approach to understanding diseases and their treatments is the most valid approach and is the best route to improving health. EBM takes this line of thinking a step further by claiming that rational practice in medicine is not just what makes sense scientifically, but what can be demonstrated to be accurate (in the case of diagnostic tests) and/or effective (in the case of therapies) in terms of actual outcomes. Outcomes of research studies become a crucial component in the justification of medical knowledge.

> 3-12: 'I think that it [EBM] at least started to have a positive impact in that it forced people to justify their knowledge claims . . . So if we want to characterize pre-EBM medicine as one where people deferred to authority without questioning where that authority came from or why that authority was the authority, then the fact that EBM at the very least forced people to have to answer the question, "Well, what's your evidence for that?", "Why are you making that decision the way you are?", "What are the grounds for that?", I think that that's actually a powerfully positive ethical outcome of evidence-based medicine.'

This can be a particularly important notion in psychiatry. Without EBM, participants believed it is difficult to challenge personal beliefs or fads in psychiatry, as there seems no basis to undermine them. In other areas of medicine, patho-physiologic knowledge can provide an avenue for challenging beliefs about diagnosis and treatment. That is, at the very least, a new idea about diagnosis or treatment ought to be consistent with scientific knowledge about patho-physiology. Because there is no such knowledge in psychiatry, it can be difficult to challenge idiosyncratic beliefs or fads. If someone were to develop a new therapy, on what basis could it be critiqued? This is as true for outlandish psychotherapies, such as primal scream therapy practised in the 1970s, as it is for mainstream psychopharmacology such as the practice of prescribing high doses of neuroleptic medications in the 1980s. EBM offers a solution to this problem. Even if new ideas cannot be challenged on the basis of their consistency with pathophysiologic knowledge, they can be challenged on the basis of effectiveness. Some interviewees from the domain of mental health saw this as a crucial ethical contribution of EBM. EBM would enable psychiatrists to protect patients from the harms of unsubstantiated interventions.

7.2.1 **Rationality and Ethics**

However, a complicated picture emerges from the interviews about how to understand the relationship between the rationality offered by evidence-based practice and ethical practice. Some participants viewed EBM as a minimal ethical standard.

> 2-7: 'Well, I think EBM gives you some kind of a guideline that maybe prevents you from doing completely stupid things. If you follow the guidelines of EBM you cannot go completely wrong.'

Others viewed EBM as ethically obligatory and even definitive of ethical practice.

> 1-1: 'I think that those physicians who are clinging to practices that have been discredited . . . that is not ethical.'

But two examples offered by the interviewees point out it can be difficult to determine what a discredited intervention is. One participant discussed the idea that non-evidence-based practice could do good.

> 1-6: 'I remember one day going to a country where everybody who comes to a physician and is a little weaker and complains of tiredness gets an intramuscular injection of vitamins. And I'm saying, "Why the hell are you doing this? I mean, you know, you have these studies showing you it has no effect?" And they say, "We are not doing any harm and they expect it and they feel better." It was a dilemma for me. I didn't argue with it. I didn't argue with what they said.'
>
> I: 'Do you think that's an ethical practice?'
>
> 1-6: 'According to them it was. According to them they were doing what's right. And who am I to judge it?'

I: 'Well, I'm asking you to judge it.'
1-6: 'If you are asking me to judge it I would say yes.'

Another participant pointed out that patients may choose a treatment option, even in the face of evidence that it would not be effective.

2-5: '. . . and one of the health economists developed what's called a decision board. So it's a piece of cardboard covered with velvet and you start off with just a circle. You've been diagnosed as having breast cancer so you put that on the board. You have two options. Option one, option two. For option one these are the possible benefits, side effects, probabilities of each. So the physician walks the patient through every decision . . . And then in essence s/he gives the board or a small copy of the board to the patient and says, "Go home. Don't make a decision now. Talk to your doctor. Talk to your husband. Come back and decide." So what this researcher wanted to look at was radiation following lumpectomy. The evidence is I think 100% in one direction. Radiation does nothing. In terms of longevity. Women do not live any longer following lumpectomy whether or not they have radiation. Whether it's due to the fact that by the time they get to radiation it's too late or whatever positive effects radiation has is counteracted by the negative cardio-toxic effect, whatever. The evidence is clear. [The researcher] went through the board with many, many women. Every single one of them wanted radiation.'

This participant went on to explain that it could be ethical to offer treatments with little demonstrated effectiveness in these types of circumstances. What these participants were highlighting is that evidence-based practice could be ethical but sometimes non-evidence-based practice could also be ethical. In these examples, what seemed to make non-evidence-based practice ethical was an endorsement of broadly shared cultural values about what should happen in a good health care encounter (see the quotation from participant 1-6) and the moral duty to offer treatment options for potentially life-threatening illnesses (see the quotation from participant 2-5). Both examples imply that it is rational to attend to patients' underlying expectations and hopes, and that pursuing the greatest good in terms of improved health outcomes is not the only goal of ethical clinical practice.

7.2.2 **Does EBM Dehumanize Practice?**

Some of the interviewees identified ways in which evidence-based practice could be unethical. First, they feared that it inappropriately restricted patient choice. A second and related point was that EBM dehumanized practice, both because it is a highly technical mode of working and because it necessarily requires the privileging of population-derived data in application to individuals whose needs and circumstances might be very different from population averages.

> 3-10: 'I think those who are relying solely or predominantly on published evidence may actually impede ethical practice for a couple of reasons. One is that ethical practice is best practice and I'm not convinced that they're practicing optimal medicine. And from an ethical standpoint, if you agree that the practice of medicine is focused on doing best for the individual patient at hand as opposed to public health, right? . . . where we're more interested in effecting benefit across a population—if you really believe that a physician's duty is focused on the individual patient at hand then I think oftentimes evidence-based medicine practice as we defined in the latter cases can do the patient a disservice. You're not treating them as an individual, right? . . . if you're just trying to apply the results of population-based clinical research to individuals, you're in some ways devaluing their individualism . . . by saying what distinguishes them from other patients is not important enough to influence that decision. To me that has an ethical implication.'

The implication is that rational practice may have to include other considerations beside research data. The notion that rational practice is ethical practice is preserved by these examples, but what constitutes rational practice is more broadly construed than in EBM.

This idea may help to explain the ambivalence about the use of EBM in the context of resource allocation of health services. Resource allocation takes place in all health systems, implicitly or explicitly, as the demand for services and interventions almost always exceeds the supply. Trying to allocate any health resource results in winners and losers, as there is rarely a service that nobody needs and everyone agrees can be eliminated. Resource allocation means that someone will go without something that she perceives she needs.

A rational decision about the allocation of a resource will take into account whether an intervention works in achieving its intended purpose, but there may be many other considerations such as opportunity cost, acceptability, or burden of suffering on those who will go without, to name just a few. Ethical resource allocation should be rational but rationality includes more elements than research data. When experts in the United Kingdom oppose the curtailment of patient choice in resource allocation decisions, they are perhaps suggesting that patient choice ought to be an important consideration in rational and ethical resource allocation. When experts in the United States support the use of EBM in resource allocation, they are perhaps criticizing the use of irrational considerations in such decisions, such as individual income (those who can afford to pay for health services will receive them).

7.2.3 **Flexible EBM**

Many participants understood adherence to EBM as falling along a spectrum. At one extreme one could adhere slavishly by trying to apply every detail gleaned from research studies in the clinic, while at the other one could be flexible, adopting the broad principles of practice identified by well-conducted research studies. Some viewed this type of flexibility as crucial, because rigid or blind adherence to EBM would fail to take into account the kinds of considerations (expectations, choice, etc.) discussed above, and this failure would impede rather than promote ethical practice. However, the notion of rigid versus flexible EBM opens up questions about what counts as evidence-based practice. Who gets to decide when and how to be flexible? At what point does flexible EBM simply stop being EBM? And if one has to be flexible in order to practise ethically, is evidence-based practice really ethical practice?

7.3 **Conclusions: The Enriched Ethics of EBM**

The experts I interviewed offered their views on the relationship between ethical values and EBM. Naturally, they did not raise every issue I discussed in Chapter 6. But putting the two together, we can construct a new version of the ethics of EBM compared to the ethics of literal EBM portrayed in Chapter 6. Figure 7.1 depicts this comparison.

EBM offers an approach to clinical practice that privileges certain types of research data in making decisions about what interventions to offer in practice. This approach is supported by an underlying ethical mandate. My exploration of experts' views about the ethics of EBM suggests that EBM developers do not see ethical values as intrinsic to the knowledge-producing and knowledge-translating activities of EBM, but view EBM as a neutral tool, only vulnerable to ethical values being exerted from the outside (such as from industry). Mental health experts and philosophers disagree. Evidence is not value-free—it is produced within specific economic, political, and ethical contexts and the interpretation of evidence will serve to favour certain theories about health, disease, illness, and disability and the assumptions and values they carry. EBM's activities, both its goals and methods, are bound up with the pursuit of health, including the moral dimension of that concept.

In psychiatry, more than any other area of medicine, the story the professional community tells about how to diagnose and treat mental illness is also a story about what mental illness is, and this implies ethical values about responsibility and blameworthiness (or lack thereof), both for having an illness and for what the person chooses to do about it. If evidence is not value-free, a practice based on evidence cannot be value-free. The real question is which values

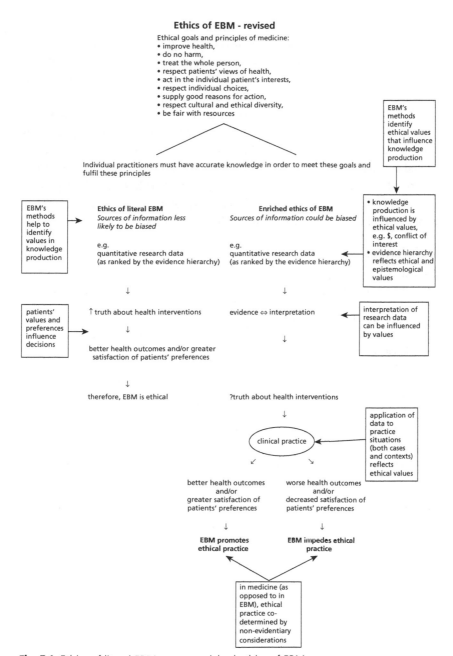

Fig. 7.1 Ethics of literal EBM versus enriched ethics of EBM.

does it privilege, and do we agree with them? Chapter 6 discussed the idea that EBM is guided ethically by a constrained utilitarianism. The experts quoted in Chapter 7 pointed out that even if we do support the values of EBM, ethical practice is rational practice, and rational practice includes considerations that lie beyond what is prioritized in EBM (research data) and what is considered good by EBM's utilitarianism (improved health outcomes and satisfaction of patients' preferences). EBM may be ethically utilitarian, but ethical practice is not. Ethical practice is determined by its own criteria. Nevertheless, the experts hinted at the idea that there is an interpretation of EBM—not the literal EBM described its authoritative texts—that is consistent with, or can be a part of, ethical psychiatric practice. What is that interpretation? And what does it say about literal EBM? Chapter 8 discusses these questions.

References

ClinicalTrials.gov™ (2005), 'Cardiac Arrhythmia Suppression Trial (CAST)' [website] <http://clinicaltrials.gov/ct2/show/study/NCT00000526?show_desc=Y#desc> accessed 13 November 2013.

Evidence-Based Medicine Working Group (1992), 'Evidence-based medicine: a new approach to teaching the practice of medicine', *Journal of the American Medical Association*, **268**: 2420–5.

Gerber, A. and Lauterbach, K. W. (2005), 'Evidence-based medicine: why do opponents and proponents use the same arguments?', *Health Care Analysis*, **13**: 59–71.

Hope, T. (2002), 'Evidence-based patient choice and psychiatry', *Evidence-Based Mental Health*, **5**: 100–1.

Parker, M. (2001), 'The ethics of evidence-based patient choice', *Health Expectations*, **4**: 87–91.

Sackett, D. L., Rosenberg, W. M. C., Gray, J. A. M., Haynes, R. B., and Richardson, W. S. (1996), 'Evidence-based medicine: what it is and what it isn't', *British Medical Journal*, **312**: 71–2.

Timmermans, S. and Berg, M. (2003), *The gold standard: the challenge of evidence-based medicine* (Philadelphia: Temple University Press).

Chapter 8

Is evidence-based psychiatric practice ethical?

8.1 The Dream of a Value-Free Psychiatry

From the late nineteenth century onwards, psychiatric researchers believed they would eventually be able to identify the pathophysiology underlying mental disorders. Over the decades theories have come and gone, but in the absence of the sought-after pathology, psychiatry continues to be dogged by criticisms that moral judgements, rather than scientific knowledge, form the basis of psychiatric diagnosis and treatment. In light of this problem, the pursuit of biological (value-free) markers of disease remains the holy grail of psychiatry. In the last generation the profession has been heavily involved in reframing mental disorder as brain disease; encouraging investment in research of the neurobiological basis of mental illness; developing ties with industry to foster psychopharmaceutical research; and moving psychiatric practice away from primary care towards an expert-consultant model, in which the psychiatrist sees patients once or infrequently, offering recommendations to another provider who carries them out.

There are, of course, many possible motivations that lie behind these actions: hospitals and universities seeking greater financial resources, researchers anxious to advance their careers, governments who want to show voters that they fund cutting-edge medical research and innovation, patients who seek social legitimacy for their suffering, and more. But in this mix of motivations there are also the insecurities of psychiatrists: scrutinized by insurers who do not wish to pay for their services and under pressure from other health care providers who argue they can do an equally good, if not better, job. If only psychiatric disorders had convincing, clear biological bases—single-gene defects, specific hormonal deficiencies, or pathognomonic structural abnormalities— psychiatrists could realize their dream of a value-free psychiatry and bring an end to the debates about the ethical legitimacy of psychiatric practice.

When the opportunity arose, psychiatrists seized upon evidence-based medicine (EBM), which advances the hierarchy of evidence as an objective standard to judge the validity of knowledge claims. EBM offers scientific validation of psychiatric interventions, a way of showing which psychiatric treatments really work to treat mental disorders. Although this does not end the search for a biological basis of mental disorder, it at least offers a partial response to critics of psychiatry's ethics. If psychiatrists apply evidence to treatment decisions, they are following the dictates of science, not moral judgement.

However, any methodology contains within it a valuation of what it can study using its procedures. In the case of health research, these values cannot be divorced from ethical values about what kinds of suffering are worth knowing about, worth intervening in, and under what circumstances. Furthermore, the methods of EBM construe mental disorder in a particular way, emphasizing certain aspects of mental experience and de-emphasizing others. When EBM directs psychiatrists' attention towards one kind of problem and away from another, it cannot help but be making an ethical judgement about who deserves care and treatment and who does not; about which kinds of problems are worth expending health care resources on and which are not. EBM carries its own ethical judgements and thus cannot be value-free. The real question for psychiatrists is whether EBM's values offer psychiatry a better vision of ethical practice than what preceded it.

8.2 The Scope of EBM

Chapters 6 and 7 explored the ethics of EBM—namely, the ethical values and the theories to which EBM seems to be committed, and the relationship between evidence-based practice and ethical practice. In Chapter 6 I argued that EBM justifies itself by making a link between the best knowledge, improved health outcomes, and ethically good practice. This link is particularly important to psychiatrists. The version of psychiatry's history most commonly found in the popular imagination characterizes the interventions of the past as coercive, even abusive, while simultaneously portraying psychiatry as unscientific. According to this view, it is the unscientific status of psychiatry that makes it unethical (Ghaemi 2009: 249). Therefore, if psychiatry has an inadequate scientific basis, on what grounds—ask the critics—are psychiatrists given a professional monopoly in the care of the mentally ill and the legal powers to enforce their treatments?

In *Ethics and evidence-based medicine: fallibility and responsibility in clinical science*, Goodman, like some of my interviewees, ties ethical practice to rational practice and argues that evidence-based practice is the best model of rational practice we have (2003: 129–40). Put this way, EBM offers psychiatrists their best hope for combating the portrayal of psychiatric knowledge as unscientific and psychiatric practice as unethical. However, this justification for EBM can be questioned in light of the numerous challenges that have been made to EBM's epistemological assumption of offering privileged access to the most valid information about health care interventions. Moreover, as we saw in Chapters 4 and 5, given the nature of psychiatric disorders and their treatments, EBM might not apply well to psychiatry and might therefore not be able to improve its scientific basis. If it cannot improve its scientific basis, it cannot improve its ethical basis. In Chapter 7, the interviewees pointed to another problem faced by those who want to strengthen the ethics of psychiatric practice through EBM. Ethical practice—even with access to valid and reliable research data—must take into account features that are not considered under EBM, and it therefore extends beyond evidence-based practice. To borrow Goodman's language, ethical practice is rational practice, but rational practice encompasses more than what is offered by EBM.

But does EBM even claim to offer a framework for ethical practice? Is ethical practice something that it was ever intended to cover? It turns out that these are difficult questions to answer because of the expansion of the concept of EBM over the last 20 years. In its infancy, EBM was limited to an approach to understanding and interpreting clinical research studies in order to inform decisions to use diagnostic tests, prescribe treatments, anticipate harms, and prognosticate. Over the ensuing years, the critical analyses of EBM have motivated EBM's authors to include more than just the application of critical appraisal to clinical decisions, thereby expanding its boundaries. For example, in subsequent editions, both *Users' guides* and *Evidence-based medicine* were revised to include consideration of patients' values and preferences alongside evidence (Guyatt et al. 2008; Straus et al. 2011). EBM includes physicians' values in decision-making through its commitment to shared decision-making. Satisfying patients' preferences is now an independent goal. The definition of EBM has also been expanded to include consideration of cost. In short, consideration of the ethical values of patients, physicians, and payers are all key components of EBM.

EBM is an approach to clinical practice that starts with patients presenting problems and ends after decisions have been made, all while considering cost and patients' and physicians' values. While this may not describe everything that happens in clinical practice, it certainly includes a substantial portion of it. If EBM offers a comprehensive—but not a complete—model of clinical practice, what aspects of practice are not explicitly covered? These might include interpersonal issues, such as personality conflicts between doctors and patients, or medico-legal determinations to hospitalize certain patients involuntarily. Do EBM's authors intend that EBM can potentially handle these issues by recourse to research data—for example, by doing research studies about interventions that identify and resolve personality conflicts? Or do the authors mean that some other model of practice or some other practice-guiding field will explain how to handle them—for example, involuntarily hospitalization of mentally ill people should be based on legal tests for risk of dangerous behaviour rather than on research evidence about the effectiveness of involuntary hospitalization?

EBM's texts provide no direct answers to these questions. If EBM is only intended to be a partial model of practice in which some clinical and ethical questions lie beyond its scope, on what grounds do we decide which questions are for EBM and which are not? To follow the involuntary hospitalization example, if several high-quality meta-analyses supported the assertion that people who are involuntarily hospitalized for schizophrenia have worse mental health outcomes, suffer more relapses, are more disabled, or are less satisfied, on what grounds would EBM proponents continue to view this as a question of law and ethics rather than one of research evidence? On the other hand, if EBM's authors acknowledge that some clinical or ethical questions lie beyond the purview of EBM, where does that end? All we know is that, at present, EBM tries to guide a very substantial portion of the activities of clinical practice, while avoiding this larger question of its scope.

If the ethics of EBM cannot serve as an overall framework for addressing some or many or most ethical questions in psychiatry then what gaps does it leave? What other approach or method should psychiatrists draw upon to fill these gaps and how might these models interact with EBM? What role does this leave for EBM and what is its real contribution to psychiatry? The rest of this chapter will discuss these questions.

8.3 **What does Ethical Psychiatric Practice Look Like?**

In Chapter 7 the Interviewees' comments showed that whatever EBM is in theory, it is ultimately a living practice whose nature can only be exposed fully when viewed in the context of actual clinical care. They discussed various clinical circumstances in which the evidence offered by EBM ran counter to what patients wanted or expected or what clinicians thought was needed. In order to practise ethically in these situations, the individual practitioner had to draw upon other principles, including the primacy of individual choice, the ethical importance of offering treatment options in terminal or serious illness, and respect for cultural diversity and local context.

Of course, as a whole, medical practice is shaped by moral guidance manifest in additional sources including professional codes of ethics, the policies of regulatory authorities, institutional policies, legislation, and jurisprudence. The theoretical basis of these sources of guidance is pluralistic and include consequentialist, deontological, virtue motivations. Yet even with these various sources, psychiatry continues to struggle with particular ethical problems that are not easily addressed either by recourse to existing ethical resources or by recourse to EBM. These include the social marginalization of mentally ill people, and the negative impact of the power imbalance between psychiatrists and patients in clinical care. By offering a seemingly sound scientific basis for psychiatric practice, psychiatrists had hoped that EBM would succeed by putting psychiatric illness on an equal footing with other diseases (thereby responding to the marginalization concern). By demonstrating that its treatments are effective, the concern about power could also be addressed—at least in part—because psychiatrists could claim that involuntary measures were not merely expressions of power but were truly needed to achieve proven therapeutic aims.

However, the ethics of EBM has not been able to help psychiatrists resolve these clinical ethical issues. What alternative approaches can practitioners bring to bear upon them? The field of psychiatry has a tradition of advocating models or visions of practice that give voice to its ethical and intellectual commitments. Here I will discuss three, all developed by psychiatrists or writers closely connected to psychiatry.[1] The first is George Engel's biopsychosocial model, which predates EBM (1977; 1979). Although Engel was mostly concerned about the problem of conceptualizing psychiatric disorders using the biomedical paradigm, he argues that all areas of medicine can benefit by re-thinking the basic assumptions of the nature of disease. The second is Patrick Bracken and Phillip Thomas' postpsychiatry, which the authors say is not a model but a critique of modernism in psychiatry (2001; 2005). Nevertheless, by noting what they critique in psychiatry we can get a glimpse of their preferred vision of practice. Among other issues, they take aim at evidence-based psychiatry. The third is Bill Fulford's values-based practice (2004; 2011). Fulford originally developed the model to apply to the domain of mental health, but believes it applies to all of medicine. He supports EBM and argues that values-based practice works in concert with EBM.

---

[1] There are several other approaches to clinical practice but these come from other specialties or domains, such as patient-centred medicine (family medicine, Canada), relationship-centred care (medical education, USA), and person-centred medicine (all of medicine, Europe).

8.3.1 **The Biopsychosocial Model**

Engel's paper on the biopsychosocial model (1977), still a classic work in psychiatry, articulated a comprehensive view of illness and disease as multiply determined, dynamic, and holistic, encompassing both the patient's experience of illness and the biological aspects of disease. He compared his approach to the standard biomedical perspective, in which disease is viewed as resulting from causal mechanisms operating in linear fashion at a molecular level within the individual organism. The model has had a profound influence on psychiatric practice to the present day. For example, the Royal College of Physicians and Surgeons of Canada identifies the biopsychosocial model as the framework to guide all instruction in psychiatry and makes clear that teachers are to instruct in accordance with this model (2007: 2).

Engel's model was influenced by systems theory. He viewed the sick individual as one component of a larger system that extended all the way from the whole population to subatomic particles. According to Engel, doctors cannot understand illness at one level without considering the implications for other levels in the system (although not all are relevant all the time). He was concerned that a reductionist model of disease orientated medical attention to the causal mechanisms at minute levels, while neglecting larger parts of the system. This is dehumanizing to patients and leads to worse (less effective, less compassionate) care, in that it privileges biological aspects of disease while ignoring social, psychological, and cultural aspects of illness. Such an approach can also be unscientific, by failing to develop a scholarly understanding of the psychosocial elements of disease and of practice. An additional implication of the biomedical view is that it denigrates the skills of the professionals who address psychosocial problems. Anyone with common sense can address psychosocial problems but only the scientifically educated physician can understand and treat disease (Engel 1979).

Engel's articulation of the model in 1977 preceded the McMaster group's first publication of the 'Reader's guides' series[2] in the *Canadian Medical Association Journal* by only a few years (see Section 2.1). In a sense, both found fault in the same place—namely, with the biomedical model. Engel believed that, by prioritizing pathophysiology, the biomedical model distracted physicians from the important psychosocial elements of practice that were necessary for better care, and for a better understanding of disease. The biopsychosocial model was intended to correct that. Sackett and colleagues believed that, by prioritizing

---

[2] The *Canadian Medical Association Journal*'s 'Readers' guides' series was one of the precursors to the book *Evidence-based medicine*.

pathophysiology, the biomedical model distracted physicians from the real, practice-changing implications of clinical research. The 'Readers' guides' series would contribute towards correcting that. But because many aspects of psychiatric problems and practice are resistant to measurement using the highly ranked methods of the evidence hierarchy, they tend to be ignored by researchers and funders. Thus, EBM's technical bias works to recreate the same problem that Engel identified in biomedicine. Engel's model was not intended to remedy EBM, of course, but because the biopsychosocial model formulates clinical problems in a manner that goes beyond the biomedical assumptions of medicine and of EBM,[3] it can act as a corrective for the impact technical bias has on psychiatric knowledge and patient care. A broader understanding of disease may then allow for interventions that are otherwise non-evidence-based.

8.3.2 Postpsychiatry

More recently, since the late 1990s, Bracken and Thomas, both psychiatrists (Bracken in Ireland, Thomas in the United Kingdom), have developed the idea of postpsychiatry. They apply a postmodernist perspective to the basic assumptions of contemporary psychiatry—namely, that mental illness needs to be controlled by experts, that mental illness can best be understood in a technical idiom, and (in a similar vein to Engel) that the problems of mental illness are located inside the individual rather than in systems, be they societies or cultures (Bracken and Thomas 2005: 8–11). They do not want to dismantle psychiatry; nor do they adopt an antipsychiatry stance, since they do not dismiss the reality of mental illness. Instead, they want to prioritize values, meaning, and relationships in psychiatry while making its technical aspects, like EBM, secondary (Bracken and Thomas 2001). They emphasize social aspects of madness (and recovery) and de-emphasize biological and psychological ones. They also prioritize the patient's perspective, even at the expense of the professional or scientific one. In this regard, they go further than Engel.

Bracken and Thomas developed postpsychiatry after the arrival of EBM and they critique it directly. They see evidence as value-laden, and argue that EBM privileges the values of professionals. In their vision of ethical psychiatry, the interests and experiences of users (patients) should be given greater emphasis, while the interests of professionals, as manifest in EBM, should be

---

[3] Even though proponents of EBM claim that EBM-preferred research methods does not require knowledge of pathogenesis in order to evaluate treatment effectiveness, Giacomini argues that EBM has to contain pathophysiological commitments (2009: 241–2). She maintains that it is not possible to devise intelligible research questions or studies without having plausible hypotheses based on a variety of theoretical (including pathophysiological) assumptions.

de-emphasized. Research data may be relevant to a given clinical scenario but cannot be applied until the psychiatrist first understands the meaning of the situation to the patient and her values. The authors reject the idea that EBM offers privileged access to the truth about medical interventions and, as such, view it as simply any other source of information. In postpsychiatry type of practice, clinicians might consider research data in decision-making but not assign it any particular preferential status. Postpsychiatry does not operate alongside EBM but instead would replace it, assigning a small role to the application of clinical research studies to practice questions.

8.3.3 Values-Based Practice

Fulford, also a psychiatrist in the United Kingdom, has developed the concept of values-based practice, a direct and intentional parallel to evidence-based practice (2004). His goal in developing values-based practice was to fill a gap left by evidence-based practice—namely, to provide a method for negotiating conflicts of values that can arise in the clinical encounter. In his words, values-based practice will help 'in coming to balanced judgments in individual cases [where values conflict]' (2011: 977). The values-based practice framework includes ten elements. The first four are practice skills that reflect competencies practitioners ought to have if they are to make clinical decisions in accordance with the values-based framework; the other six are claims or principles advocated by the framework. The practice skills include: 1) awareness of values; 2) reasoning about values; 3) knowledge of values and facts; and 4) communication. The six claims or principles are that: 5) services ought to be user-centred and 6) multidisciplinary; 7) evidence-based practice and values-based practice work together; 8) we only notice values when there is a problem; 9) increasing scientific knowledge increases choices, which can demonstrate divergence in values; and 10) values-based practice involves providers and users making decisions in partnership (Fulford 2011: 981).

These ten principles are meant to work in tandem with evidence-based practice, in the sense that research data should be considered alongside the values of all those involved in the clinical encounter (including those not necessarily present, such as the hospital, society, insurers, etc.). Although values-based practice places greater emphasis on the role of values in clinical practice, it stakes out a less radical position than postpsychiatry by seeking to collaborate with evidence-based practice as an equal partner, rather than relegating it to second place. Like EBM's authors, Fulford treats EBM as value-free, claiming it provides the 'facts' of medicine (2011: 981 and 984). Meanwhile, values-based practice is there to handle the values of practice, which lie outside EBM.

Fulford's view of ethical practice is one in which the values of all parties are made explicit and discussed fully and openly.

In a similar vein to what the interviewees pointed out, all three approaches highlight the idea that ethical psychiatric practice encompasses more than what EBM can tell us. They do, however, offer different solutions to fill in the gap. Engel contends that one cannot practise optimally in the absence of understanding the psychosocial dimensions of disease. His model also helps to address the problem of technical bias. A more comprehensive understanding of disease may require us to consider other types of interventions than the ones prioritized by EBM. Bracken and Thomas focus more on which parties should be involved, wanting to reduce the role and power of professionals and enhance the participation of users in their own care and the care of others. Their approach fills in the values embedded within EBM and shows how these values affect therapeutic options and decisions. Fulford contends that one cannot really practise without a process for negotiating the values held by each party. His approach addresses the issue of how to handle those interpersonal aspects of practice related to conflicts of values. These authors offer ways for psychiatry to handle the kinds of ethical considerations that arise in clinical practice, but for which EBM offers no guidance. The lasting impact of these diverse approaches will be evaluated with the passage of time.

8.4 **Responsible Knowers**

The approaches discussed in this chapter can be considered to do some of the ethical work that EBM does not have the resources to do on its own. They seek to improve the ethics of practice by focusing on better knowledge, redistributing power from professionals to users, and developing fair processes for considering values. These ideas develop and enrich the notion of ethical psychiatric practice, and show that EBM may only be able to play a limited role in psychiatric practice—more limited than its texts currently claim. But if, as I have argued in this book, EBM improves neither the knowledge nor the ethics of psychiatry, why should we want it to play any role in psychiatric practice at all?

Recall that the EBM texts are evasive on the question of its ultimate goal. In Chapter 6 I argued that EBM had two goals: improved health outcomes (implicit) and satisfying patients' preferences (explicit). However, if we look back at the fifth and final step of practising EBM—evaluation—neither of these goals is mentioned. Instead, evaluation is self-referential: has the practitioner successfully completed steps 1–4? Does this mean that the real goal of EBM is to be able to do EBM well? And if so, what does this tell us about EBM?

The original idea of critical appraisal focuses on helping the practitioner become a better knower. This entails learning certain skills but also developing certain attitudes involved in acquiring knowledge. When EBM's authors challenge practitioners to supply evidence upon which to base clinical actions, they are asking practitioners to reflect upon, and make explicit, the justification for their beliefs. By following the rules of critical appraisal, EBM offers the practitioner good reasons to draw certain types of conclusions about medical interventions. If the practitioner acts on the basis of conclusions supported by the kinds of evidence sanctioned by EBM, he is epistemically blameless, meaning that he has done what a responsible practitioner should have done. Here we see the link again between good knowledge and ethics, but this time in reference to the practitioner rather than the outcome of his actions. In fact, the responsibility to improve one's medical knowledge is a recognized ethical obligation of physicians commonly found in professional codes of ethics. For example, the Canadian Medical Association's 'Code of ethics' contains within its very first section on fundamental responsibilities the requirement that each physician 'engage in lifelong learning to maintain and improve your professional knowledge, skills and attitudes' (Canadian Medical Association 2004). Maintaining one's knowledge is ethically important because the practitioner will use that knowledge to intervene in cases of individual illness and suffering where his actions, based on these beliefs, have the potential to help or harm someone else.

As EBM has evolved, it has moved beyond the individual practitioner using critical appraisal strategies to justify her beliefs on her own. Instead, the focus is on practitioners consulting pre-appraised EBM sources—that is, those borne of a reliable, knowledge-producing procedure. EBM's authors have never been concerned about this move, even though it shifts away from the individual practitioner seeking evidence to justify her beliefs. If a practitioner consults pre-appraised sources, she can still claim to be justified in holding a belief because she followed a reliable procedure to do so. Although these are two different approaches to justifying medical knowledge, they are united by EBM's original challenge: to supply a good rationale for one's decisions and actions. This challenge is at once epistemological and ethical. What EBM seems to be asking is that practitioners be epistemically responsible for the knowledge that underlies their decisions. Now, I have argued that the responsible knower in psychiatry ought to question whether adhering to EBM really does offer valid justification for medical beliefs, because the complexity of mental disorders and their treatments resists easy measurement by the standards of EBM. I have also argued that the distortions to which the medical research literature is subject should provoke doubt in any critical thinker. If a psychiatrist adheres to the rules of EBM without taking these issues into consideration then she is vulnerable to making poor clinical decisions. This would make her epistemically and ethically blameworthy.[4]

Nevertheless, even if the application of EBM's principles cannot provide the justification of certain beliefs, EBM's charge to be judicious and explicit in the use of clinical evidence may be quite important. It can be interpreted as a call to cultivate intellectual virtues. In addition to judiciousness and explicitness, these could include open-mindedness and the capacity for debate. And, as discussed in Chapter 6, EBM also seems to encourage the cultivation of moral virtues such as conscientiousness, honesty, and courage in the face of pressure to adopt one belief over another. These moral virtues are necessary to being a responsible medical knower. Formulating EBM as a call to virtue offers a link between epistemology and ethics. Good knowing in medicine has both intellectual and ethical aspects, and being a good knower requires both intellectual and moral virtues. Thinking of EBM as having a basis in virtues may make sense of EBM's puzzling claim that the goal of EBM is to be good at EBM. Rather than interpreting the ethics of EBM along utilitarian lines it may be more fruitful to re-interpret it in virtue theory terms. That is, rather than thinking that by using its methods practitioners will achieve certain practice outcomes, it may be more accurate to construe EBM as a method for developing the capacity to be responsible knowers. Evidence-based practice may not necessarily be ethical practice, but it may offer a distinct ethical stance from which psychiatry could benefit.

8.5 **Conclusions**

Plagued by the perennial debates concerning the question of whether psychiatry is a legitimate medical discipline, psychiatrists saw EBM as a beacon of hope. Finally, they believed, there would be scientific data to substantiate the effectiveness of psychiatric treatments and, perhaps by association, the validity of psychiatric diagnoses. EBM, after all, offered itself as a route to accurate knowledge about treatments, and if psychiatrists could provide treatments that work, this would show that psychiatric practice was effective and ethical, and at least some of the ethical doubts about the field could be assuaged.

However, as we have seen in this book, EBM, the evidence hierarchy, and the prioritization of the randomized controlled trial (RCT) do not take into account the potential for profound distortions in the medical literature, which is driven

---

[4] I borrow the phrase 'epistemically blameworthy' from Freedman's paper, 'Traumatic blocking and Brandom's oversight' (2007).

to a large extent by the financial interests of private industry. Furthermore, the methods of EBM are, on the whole, poorly conceived to provide accurate and useful information concerning the problems and treatments that make up the bulk of psychiatric practice. We have good reason to doubt that adherence to the methodology of EBM will help psychiatrists to practise more effectively. Even if this were not the case, adopting an EBM approach to psychiatry dodges the truly vexing problems in psychiatric practice, many of which are ethical in nature. EBM either assumes that these issues are unproblematic (e.g. questions of diagnostic validity) or has nothing to say about them (e.g. involuntary hospitalization). The utilitarian impulses of the ethics of EBM, which seek to optimize mental health outcomes, are insufficient as a guide to ethical psychiatric practice. There are simply too many other morally relevant features to consider. Where should psychiatrists turn for guidance, if not EBM?

Perhaps the first place is back to psychiatry itself. The three approaches discussed earlier demonstrate that psychiatrists are already, and have been for some time, engaged in thinking about the moral superstructure that frames all of psychiatry. These values find their inspiration in the currents that flow through the history of modern psychiatry: in moral treatment, in the aspirations of the first biological psychiatry, in antipsychiatry, and now in the recovery movement and critical psychiatry. It remains to be seen what the next version of ethical psychiatry will look like. What is becoming increasingly clear is that it will not be realized through the lens of EBM. But paradoxically, perhaps EBM will serve as a timely reminder that, in psychiatry, the RCT will not replace the moral necessity for responsible scientific knowing.

References

Bracken, P. and Thomas, P. (2001), 'Postpsychiatry: a new direction for mental health', *British Medical Journal*, **322**: 724–7.

Bracken, P. and Thomas, P. (2005), *Postpsychiatry: mental health in a postmodern world* (Oxford: Oxford University Press).

Canadian Medical Association (2004), 'CMA code of ethics (update 2004)' [website]. <http://policybase.cma.ca/dbtw-wpd/PolicyPDF/PD04-06.pdf> accessed 9 November 2013).

Engel, G. L. (1977), 'The need for a new medical model: a challenge for biomedicine', *Science*, **196**: 129–36.

Engel, G. L. (1979), 'The biopsychosocial model and the education of health professionals', *General Hospital Psychiatry* **1**: 156–65.

Freedman, K. L. (2007), 'Traumatic blocking and Brandom's oversight', *Philosophy, Psychiatry, and Psychology*, **14**: 1–12.

Fulford, K. W. M. (2004), 'Ten principles of values-based medicine', in: Radden, J. (ed.), *The philosophy of psychiatry: a companion* (New York: Oxford University Press), 205–34.

Fulford, K.W.M. (2011), 'The value of evidence and evidence of values: bringing together values-based and evidence-based practice in policy and service development in mental health', *Journal of Evaluation in Clinical Practice*, **17**: 976–87.

Ghaemi, S. N. (2009), 'The case for, and against, evidence-based psychiatry', *Acta Psychiatrica Scandanavica*, **119**: 249–51.

Giacomini, M. (2009), 'Theory-based medicine and the role of evidence', *Perspectives in Biology and Medicine*, **52**: 234–51.

Goodman, K. W. (2003), 'Ethics and evidence', in: *Ethics and evidence-based medicine: fallibility and responsibility in clinical science* (Cambridge: Cambridge University Press), 129–40.

Guyatt, G., Rennie, D., Meade, M., and Cook, D. (eds.) (2008), *Users' guides to the medical literature: a manual for evidence-based clinical practice*, 2nd edn. (Chicago: AMA Press).

Royal College of Physicians and Surgeons of Canada (2007), 'Specific standards of accreditation for residency programs in psychiatry' [website] <http://www.royalcollege.ca/portal/page/portal/rc/public

Enter:Information by Discipline

Enter:Psychiatry

Enter: Specific Standards of Accreditation for Residency Programs (see Standard B4)> accessed 25 May 2009.

Straus, S. E., Richardson, W. S., Glasziou, P., and Haynes, R. B. (2011), *Evidence-based medicine: how to practice and teach EBM*, 4th edn. (Edinburgh: Churchill Livingstone Elsevier).

Chapter 9

Conclusions

Evidence-based medicine (EBM) is underscored by the basic ethical value to pursue health and is based on an epistemological assumption that its methods will show us which interventions achieve health most effectively. Most of the critical literature examining EBM accepts its basic value, but takes issue with this epistemological assumption. Do EBM's methods really lead us to better knowledge, specifically when it comes to clinical questions concerning treatment, harm, diagnosis, and prognosis? This body of literature suggests that there are good reasons to think that EBM is not the most accurate route to medical knowledge—particularly not for the field of psychiatry, where the nature of mental disorders and their treatment do not conform well to the demands of EBM.

Even if EBM really was a route to more accurate psychiatric knowledge, its ethics may also be inadequate for psychiatric practice. In spite of the fact that they are not acknowledged, EBM has ethical values embedded at every level: from the design of research studies through to the interpretation and dissemination of research data. Applying research data in clinical scenarios without giving attention to the assumptions about health and suffering that have been made to generate those data can be unethical. The same is true regarding blindness to the social and ethical context of knowledge production in psychiatric research. In both cases, interests and values are being masked and presented as evidence. Instead, ethical practice requires making these values explicit and negotiating rather than obscuring them.

I have argued that EBM's underlying ethical motivations are utilitarian and that utilitarianism cannot help psychiatry to resolve its ethical problems in spite of hopes from within the profession that it will. At the same time, the EBM experts I interviewed noted that ethical practice is rational practice, and insofar as EBM is rational it facilitates ethical practice. However, EBM is not the only standard for rational practice. Rational practice goes beyond EBM, which means that ethical practice also extends beyond EBM. Because ethical values necessarily play a role in determining how we understand mental disorder and how we propose to intervene, it may be rational for values to direct practice, including the option of offering and making choices that are non-evidence-based. This does not mean that we have to accept ideology and fads, but it does mean that we have to reach beyond EBM's restricted notion of evidence to responsible knowing: judiciousness, explicitness, openness, and debate. Paradoxically, it is a return to the origins of EBM that might point us in this direction.

What are the implications of these arguments? The first is that evidence-based practice is not necessarily ethical practice. While EBM focuses our attention on specific types of research questions, methods, and outcomes, it obscures the ethical values that shape its practice. Second, in view of its epistemological limitations, EBM is insufficient as a method of generating accurate psychiatric knowledge about diagnosis, treatment, harm, and prognosis. EBM is a constraining discourse, narrowing how we understand and intervene in mental disorders, which itself has significant ethical implications. EBM could even end up being a model of bad practice—in which practitioners and patients draw premature conclusions about what is best practice where there is legitimate room for debate and difference. This could be more damaging to psychiatry than other medical disciplines, since it has been plagued by controversy about the use and abuse of power since its inception.

What does this mean for psychiatry and for evidence-based psychiatry? The analysis offered in this book suggests three main conclusions. The first is that EBM, or at least evidence-based psychiatry, could be improved if it were to contract: aim to do a smaller task that would be at once more modest but also more defensible, epistemologically and ethically. In light of this, the second conclusion is that psychiatry needs to reject the constraining discourse of EBM and define the questions and methods that are appropriate to the subject material of its discipline—whether or not these are part of the subject matter of the rest of medicine. The third conclusion is that bioethical analysis offers psychiatry a helpful companion for this work. The methods and perspectives of bioethics can enable practitioners to be more aware of ethical values that pervade its practice, thereby opening up opportunities for explicit debate and dialogue within the field and with patients and policy-makers. I discuss each conclusion in turn.

9.1 **The Future of EBM: The Case for Contraction[1]**

EBM started out as critical appraisal of clinical research based on the idea of the evidence hierarchy of research methods and an optimal study design for each method on the hierarchy. The evidence hierarchy has been subject to

---

[1] I am grateful to Dr Jorge Holguin who suggested this apt turn of phrase.

philosophical criticism, but philosophers have also argued that it is defensible as a hierarchy of internal validity (LaCaze 2009), and that internal validity is defensible as a standard to judge the merits of clinical research (Howick 2011: 55). Of course, offering a strategy for assessing clinical research methods for their relative internal validity is a less compelling project than one that claims to offer a base for all of medicine. However, I have argued in this book that the expansiveness of EBM is exactly where it loses clarity and becomes less defensible. Many interviewees agreed that EBM's original focus on critical appraisal was innovative and an improvement to the ethics of practice. It was in its evolution that EBM had become an unwieldy and ill-defined concept.

When EBM is about judging the extent to which certain types of clinical research studies are able to generate accurate data about certain types of research questions, it makes sense. For clinicians to have the skills to understand and interpret these types of studies so that they can take them into consideration, debate their relative merits with colleagues, and use this process to arrive at considered judgements on how to proceed in clinical care is a reasonable part of what it means to be a skilled practitioner. For our purposes, it is also defensible ethically, as critical appraisal can contribute knowledge towards answering clinical questions whose purpose is to relieve suffering. This fits into the existing ethical framework of medical practice, leaving larger questions such as how to present information or how one deals with ethical issues regarding treatment choices to that larger framework.

However, EBM has expanded considerably, offering quantitative algorithms for factoring patients' values into clinical decision-making and including physicians' values, all while considering cost. Once it claims to cover these aspects of practice it is claiming, by stealth, to do the work that various ethical frameworks and policies are currently trying to do. Is it capable of doing this job? I have argued that it is not. EBM is largely underwritten ethically by utilitarianism, and these principles will not be able to do the ethical work that is needed in psychiatric practice. Rather, EBM's real ethical contribution lies in its emphasis on the importance of continued cultivation of intellectual and ethical virtue.

Is it possible for EBM's authors to strengthen its theoretical foundation by taking it back to basics? That is, could EBM simply return to being about relative internal validity, or could it include an expanded view of critical appraisal that systematically examined the various forces that influence (and distort) medical knowledge production, not merely a subset of biases relevant to the conduct of certain kinds of studies? Even without the participation of EBM's authors, opinion leaders in psychiatry could take up this challenge by redefining EBM, or at least critical appraisal, to fit the needs of psychiatry. At a minimum, this would involve specifying the kinds of questions that EBM is capable of answering in psychiatry, what is left out by this approach, and what is needed in order to address the other questions. Using this approach, psychiatrists (and patients) would determine what they need to know about mental disorders, rather than EBM telling them that what is worth knowing. Whether this type of revision is possible in an era where distinctions between mental health and the rest of medicine are discouraged (Insel and Quirion 2005) is uncertain.

9.2 The Future of Psychiatry: The Case for Expansion

What is the alternative to EBM? This is the question I face most often from fellow psychiatrists. In this book I have argued that psychiatry is a complex field, whose subject matter is, in many respects, distinct from that of most areas of medicine even while it remains part of medicine. Clinical psychiatry has to find a way to pursue the knowledge it needs to meet its aims—namely, to relieve mental suffering and improve the lives of the people who depend on it. Moreover, because of its controversial history, psychiatry may need to consider ethical issues that figure less in other areas of medicine. In practice, this means that psychiatrists must be able to address intellectual challenges that might seem at odds with trends in other areas of medicine. For example, psychiatrists rely heavily on subjective knowledge in diagnosing and treating mental illness. This might include patients' self-reported symptoms, one's own feelings in response to patients, and others' observations and reports. There is a paucity of knowledge about how one should optimally harness these sources of knowledge in making diagnoses, prescribing treatment, and assessing response. In other areas of medicine this line of thinking may not be of great interest, given that diagnosis is almost always made on the basis of changes to anatomical or physiological function, treatment is typically prescribed to remove or palliate this dysfunction, and the effect of treatment is evaluated by determining the extent to which the underlying deficit is corrected. However, psychiatrists cannot rely on these types of indicators and must have their own, appropriate to the fact that mental disorders cannot be assessed and treated in this way.

The current approach in psychiatry is to make its procedures as much like procedures in other areas of medicine as possible—for example, instead of having to rely only on self-report of symptoms, objective symptom-rating scales are developed to use in tandem or instead. But this gets the solution wrong. Psychiatry will be better off developing tools, approaches, and research that does justice to the complexity of its subject material rather than making it as intelligible as possible through the medical, or evidence-based medical, idiom. This will require an expansion of psychiatric thinking to encompass more topics and more methods than it currently employs. Such pluralism might be at once less medical but more scientific. Practitioners and patients alike could benefit from a deeper understanding of how one human, by means of detailed personal engagement, comes to help in the healing of another.

9.3 **Bioethics and Psychiatry: The Need for Continued Engagement**

Bioethics has contributed to reflection in psychiatry about whether some of its contentious practices, such as involuntary hospitalization, are morally justifiable. Medicine is an ethical venture and psychiatry even more so, given that the field deals with some of the most puzzling and difficult problems that humans face. Bioethical analysis can go further than it has, and provide psychiatry with assistance further upstream by identifying and questioning the values that are at play in its basic tasks. The question is not whether values are at work in psychiatric practice, but whose values and why? A major aspect of the public and professional impression of EBM is the extent to which evidence can somehow determine moral judgement, or even does away with the need for moral judgement—a welcome development for many clinicians vexed by ethically difficult clinical situations where values can be diverse.

One of the most important contributions of bioethical analysis is to show how values are part of EBM, evidence-based psychiatry, and indeed of evidence itself. EBM cannot be viewed as a neutral mediator between competing values but must be seen as contributing certain values. This development encourages EBM users to be aware of values at every level, including at the level of the basic information we provide to patients. Opening up these conversations as discussions about values permits a natural evolution towards patients as true collaborators in determining the trajectory of their care.

A promising area for further work in ethics and EBM/evidence-based psychiatry is to investigate the interface of evidence and ethical values in clinical practice. The theoretical portrayal (literal EBM) of values in evidence-based practice is essentially of patients' values as a gatekeeper, determining which interventions will be undertaken and which will be avoided. In this book I have identified a far greater role for ethical values in evidence-based practice. How does a practitioner integrate these values with the principles of evidence-based practice? Does the particular nature of mental disorders and what is known about them present specific ethical challenges in attempting to apply the principles of EBM? These questions would ideally be addressed by prolonged field observations of clinical practice and interviews with practitioners and patients.

In the meantime, EBM in whatever form is unlikely to be going anywhere. The field of psychiatry must determine for itself whether it will continue to be swept along in this latest chapter in the history of medical ideas or whether it will heed EBM's most important advice: to be conscientious and judicious in the use of evidence.

References

Howick, J. (2011), *The philosophy of evidence-based medicine* (Chichester: Wiley-Blackwell).

LaCaze, A. (2009), 'Evidence-based medicine must be . . .', *Journal of Medicine and Philosophy*, **34**: 509–27.

Insel, T.R. and Quirion, R. (2005), 'Psychiatry as a clinical neuroscience discipline', *Journal of the American Medical Association*, **294**: 2221–4.

Appendix 1

Methods for the empirical (interview) project

In the first phase of researching this book I examined the primary texts concerning evidence-based medicine (EBM) and the academic literature on this topic. This review drew my attention to some of the key conceptual and ethical issues as well as the unanswered questions facing EBM and evidence-based psychiatry. The first phase of the project also allowed me to provide a provisional analysis of the ethics of EBM as elucidated from its key texts. This analysis informed the second, empirical stage of research, which involved interviews with EBM experts about their understanding of the ethics of EBM and evidence-based psychiatry. I interviewed three groups of participants: group 1 consisted of people who have been involved in the development of EBM; group 2 consisted of practitioners working in mental health who are involved in the implementation and debate about the use of EBM in mental health practice; and group 3 consisted of scholars who had investigated philosophical or ethical aspects of EBM. The participants' viewpoints clarified and extended what was found in the EBM texts. I was then able to analyse the interviews to re-develop an enriched version of the ethical commitments of EBM.

Why was an empirical investigation of this kind necessary? Typically, what is ethical has been the domain of philosophically orientated bioethical analysis, while a description of what people believe to be ethical falls within the scope of sociology or anthropology. Shouldn't an ethics investigation aim to unravel the ethical aspects (theories, principles, values) at play at the conceptual level, independent of what any interviewee thinks they might be? After all, an interviewee's description of the ethics of EBM is just that—a description—which does not mean that those *are* the ethical commitments of EBM.

The ethics of EBM and evidence-based psychiatry could not be adequately investigated without an empirical phase for two reasons. First, EBM is more than a concept or theory—it is also a model of practice. This means that it cannot be fully understood unless it is examined as it functions in practice by those who attempt to implement and use it. Writing about the Russian context, Geltzer's (2009) qualitative analysis of 35 interviews concerning the uptake of

EBM in that country aptly demonstrates how the application of the theory of EBM is practice-context specific. Second, the theory of EBM is underdeveloped, and aspects such as its ethics are mostly implied rather than stated. Thus, its ethical commitments are more completely understood by asking those individuals who have been most closely involved in its development, implementation, and critique to clarify and extend what is found in the texts—including what they assume and interpret from what is written and not written. It is the iterative process between what is contained in the written sources about EBM, how users understand those sources, and how they practise EBM and evidence-based psychiatry that more fully explicates its ethics. As a result, both textual and human sources were needed to identify the ethics of EBM and evidence-based psychiatry.

A1.1 **Research Tradition**

EBM is itself an approach to how to conduct and evaluate research, but one has to step entirely outside its epistemological framework in order to research it. This is because the research strategies endorsed by EBM as being the most valid (such as meta-analyses and randomized controlled trials (RCTs)) would not allow one to investigate the questions that form the focus of this project—questions that are descriptive and non-quantitative rather than experimental. Thus, I turned to qualitative approaches that offer systematic methods of gathering and analysing non-quantitative data.

The empirical component of this project used the qualitative approach of case study (Stake 1995; Yin 2003). Such an approach has been employed across disciplines (Yin 2003: 1) and there are several texts that describe how to conduct case study research. Of these, two authors are acknowledged as being leading experts in this method: Robert E. Stake and Robert K. Yin (Lohfeld, personal communication 2004). Yin's definition of the case study is 'an empirical enquiry that investigates a contemporary phenomenon within its real-life context, especially when the boundaries between phenomenon and context are not clearly evident' (Yin 2003: 13). This is certainly true when considering the question of how practitioners describe the ethics of evidence-based psychiatry. The specific principles, rules, and values they might identify are likely to be embedded within the larger scheme of clinical practice and, even more broadly, within the professional, cultural, and ethical norms of the medical community. Stake defines a case study as a research strategy intended to investigate 'objects' (people, institutions, events) 'bounded' in place and time (Stake 1995: 2). It is less apparent that the ethics of evidence-based psychiatry are bounded in this manner, as they are not defined by discrete temporal or geographical parameters.

While case study research emerged from the social sciences, the field of bio-ethics has more recently adopted it. The advent of empirical bioethics—the attempt to describe the moral world rather than philosophize about it—has sent bioethicists searching for appropriate strategies to investigate their topics. Qualitative approaches, particularly the case study method, have been welcomed by bioethicists wanting to draw upon empirical data that preserve the complexity and meaningfulness of ethical problems (Bell et al. 2004; Martin et al. 2003a; 2003b). Thus, the choice of the case study method for a bioethics research project is particularly fitting.

At the same time, there can be concerns about using this type of method for the purpose that I intended. A major issue in any qualitative research is how one can generalize (transfer) findings from one group of sources, such as a group of interviewees, to others. For example, what one group of participants report in one study is not representative—nor is it intended to be—of what a larger group of people believe, including those with similar characteristics to the participants. Thus, both the philosophy and the design of any qualitative approach limit the possibility of drawing conclusions applicable to a larger universe.[1] Using the authoritative EBM texts as a source of data addresses to some extent this question about transferability. While the participants were only speaking for themselves, they were doing so in reference to *Evidence-based medicine* and *Users' guides*, which are the original, authoritative descriptions of EBM. The participants (and, therefore, others within the larger medical and research communities) have an agreed-upon source for their views, meaning they can at least agree on the terms of the debate. The extent to which the debate can then apply to one's own context can be assessed by the reader.

A1.2 **Methods**

In this project I was guided by methodological precepts articulated by Stake and Yin—at times drawing from Stake, at others from Yin. While Stake's approach may be viewed as constructivist and Yin's as post-positivist, the two authors share some views (e.g. definitions of case study research, the importance of guiding research questions) and endorse specific techniques (e.g. the need for multiple sources of data) that are philosophically compatible

---

[1] This concern is of particular importance within the quantitative experimental traditions, where the overall purpose of research is to obtain generalizable conclusions. Qualitative researchers have a somewhat different concern about 'transferability'—the ability of one's project's data to be applicable to other participants or groups of interest (rather than population in general). I will use the term 'transferability' rather than 'generalizability' as it is more appropriate for the aims of this project.

in combination. Why the need for combining methods? Case study methods are in evolution, with leading exponents often covering different subjects or aspects of enquiry. For example, Yin recommends specific techniques designed to enhance rigour, such as the chain of evidence. A chain of evidence makes transparent the researcher's analytic choice points and the reasoning behind her choices. Stake, on the other hand, does not develop a detailed notion of rigour. Nevertheless, there is nothing within Stake's approach, or within a constructivist epistemology more generally, that would eschew this technique.

The participants agreed to give individual interviews about EBM, evidence-based psychiatry, and ethics. Most informants lived and worked in Canada, the United States, and the United Kingdom while the project was underway. Because of the geographical distance between us, some participants were interviewed by telephone. I selected the interviewees through a combination of several sampling strategies. Politically important case sampling, which identifies people considered to be important or highly knowledgeable about the topic (Creswell 1998: 119), was used to solicit the participation of several potential key informants from each of the three groups. Chain sampling, in which current participants identified other knowledgeable people, was also used to identify other potential respondents. These two sampling techniques were used until informational saturation had been achieved—that is, the point at which there are no new data exemplifying analytic categories (Creswell 1998: 243). This stands in contrast to theoretical saturation, in which the researcher returns to the field in order to gather further data from purposefully selected sources in order to test the emerging theory. By the project's end, I had interviewed 33 participants: nine in group 1, 11 in group 2, and 13 in group 3. Following each interview, I completed a 'post-mortem form' that allowed me to reflect on content and process of the interview, including my own reactions to it. In keeping with the iterative aspect of qualitative data collection and analysis, the post-mortem reflections enabled me to modify the interview guide in light of previous participants' answers and suggestions.

Yin identifies three principles of data collection (2003: 97) including: 1) the use of multiple sources of data in order to achieve evidentiary convergence;[2] 2) creating a case study database (compiling collected data in a retrievable, reviewable form so that it is accessible to outside scrutiny); and 3) maintaining a chain of evidence documenting methodological choice points and the rationales behind them. I used multiple sources of data in the form of three

----

[2] Stake also endorses this principle.

distinct interview groups in order to develop a multi-perspectival understanding of the ethics of evidence-based psychiatry. The project's database consists of all interview transcripts and the coding scheme, with definitions of each code along with corresponding excerpts from the text for each code. I also compiled a methodological decision trail, my reflexive memos, and my interview post-mortem forms into an electronic file. This document revealed my own attitudes and values, which inevitably contribute to and shape the research process and findings.

A1.3 **Analytic Procedures**

A1.3.1 **Interpretive Framework**

I drew upon the internal critique of science to organize and analyse the data (Tiles 1996: 220). This group of critiques argues that even if one sets aside the contextual values that frame science (and medical research), there remain values that are constitutive of those endeavours. Whatever objective standard is used to determine whether results, laws, or theories are true or false, this same standard must also be tied to a normative notion of how this should be achieved. This view does not require that the results of scientific study ought to be rejected as false, but recognizes that any standard that favours one set of results, or interpretation of results, must yield results that are partial and are 'conditioned by interests and values' (Tiles 1996: 224). These values are tied to the goals of science through both specific methods and specific desired outcomes.

I borrowed from the internal critique of science to inform my examination of the interview data about the ethics of EBM and evidence-based psychiatry in three specific ways. First, my investigation of the ethical commitments of EBM was underscored by the point that medical research about a particular intervention or health outcome is only ever a partial view of it. Some of the gap is filled in by our views of what constitutes health—which is ultimately an ethical view about how health contributes to living a good life. This is particularly clear in the case of psychiatry: our notions of mental health are dependent on what we think are good subjective experiences. In my analysis, I was interested in what versions of mental health might be promoted by EBM and what versions might be neglected. Second, the recourse to methodology via the evidence hierarchy is a way of establishing an objective standard for identifying valid versus invalid data. This standard can be tied to certain ethical values about the worthiness of disorders, treatments, effects, and suffering. Third, internal values of EBM in particular may converge, diverge, or operate in parallel with values that already animate medicine and psychiatry. I was, therefore, interested to know how participants viewed this intersection of values.

A1.3.2 **Data Analytic Techniques**

Drawing upon the editing style of data organization (Crabtree and Miller 1999: 21–2), I began by examining the transcripts without a set of predefined codes. Using the qualitative data management software package HyperResearch, I developed codes (words or phrases) as I read the text—codes which were attached to text segments (phrases, statements, or paragraphs) in the transcripts. The codes were listed and defined in a modifiable electronic codebook. The codebook evolved by comparing prior and current applications of codes. Therefore, codes were added, dropped, and merged depending on the review of later transcripts. The emerging codebook served an additional iterative function, informing me about the need for modifications to the interview guides and propositions.

Once the codebook was complete, I grouped many codes into smaller numbers of supra-codes, which captured themes in the interviews. These supra-codes facilitated pattern recognition of themes within and between participant groups. I was also able to identify themes exclusive to one or two groups versus all three groups. Using the data, I was able to refine the earlier framework describing the ethics of evidence-based psychiatry. The emerging interpretation was also emailed to agreeable participants with a request for feedback about any errors, omissions, or further considerations. The feedback I received did not require changes to the analysis.

A1.3.3 **Rigour**

In this project, rigour was established according to how well the research met credibility, fittingness, and auditability, the three criteria of rigour described in the literature concerning qualitative research (Sandelowski 1986: 29–33). Yin recommends similar criteria for rigour used in quantitative research, including internal validity, external validity, construct validity, and reliability (Yin 2003: 34). Although Yin argues that these criteria are applicable to any kind of social research, I have chosen to use Sandelowski's criteria. Yin's criteria have very particular meanings within quantitative approaches, and in using the same terms there is a danger that qualitative techniques will be expected to fulfil these criteria in the same manner. Using altogether different terminology emphasizes the need to judge qualitative research on its own terms, bearing in mind its specific capabilities and limitations.

Credibility refers to the ability of a research project to present 'faithful descriptions or interpretations' of experience (Sandelowski 1986: 30). Developing credibility was built into the methods of the project by sending summaries of the emerging interpretations for each group to all participants (all participants wished to receive these summaries). I also sent a copy of the individual transcript to any participant who wished to receive it (about half of the participants wanted their transcripts). I asked them to send me feedback about any errors or omissions on my part, a process known as member-checking. Member-checking contributes to credibility by allowing participants to ensure that the data and interpretation accurately reflect their views. Fittingness refers to the match between the data and the themes and categories developed in the study. I strove to achieve this by ensuring that each finding is linked to the raw data, and that higher-level abstractions are supported by actual quotes or excerpts from transcripts. Auditability refers to the transparency of the research decision-making process. I justified overall methodological choices, as well as specific data analytic issues, in a chain of evidence so that these could be examined and replicated by others if warranted. I exposed my attitudes and beliefs in research memos and interview post-mortem forms. Finally, I saved the anonymized computer files of the transcripts. These will be kept for ten years following the completion of the study, in accordance with best practice in qualitative research.

A1.4 **Ethical Oversight**

The major ethical considerations for this project are those that are traditionally identified in human subject research—specifically, obtaining informed consent including the entitlement to withdraw, providing confidentiality in gathering and storing data, ensuring anonymity in reporting data, and providing participants with feedback concerning the conclusions of the research. No participant chose to withdraw from the study or to withdraw any data.

The protocol for this project was reviewed and approved by the University of Toronto Research Ethics Board (Health Sciences). The protocol adhered to the basic requirements of ethical research in accordance with the Canadian Tri-Council Policy on Research Involving Human Subjects.

A1.5 **Limitations**

There are several potential limitations of the empirical project that should be mentioned. First, as in all qualitative research, there is a limit to the extent to which the findings can be transferred to individuals in different contexts. In keeping with the parameters of case study research, these findings should be considered to be consistent with the dominant ideas about EBM, evidence-based psychiatry, and ethics at the time the data were collected (2008).

The ideas and analysis reported here are not intended to be representative of all views about EBM. At the same time, I did interview several leading participants in the growing debate about EBM; therefore, I was able to include many of the key English language viewpoints. Further, I asked all participants if they would suggest other potential participants and I was able to interview several of them. However, I only conducted interviews in English with fluent English speakers. Therefore, any major contributors to the critical debates about EBM who do not speak or publish in English would not be included.

A second limitation is that these viewpoints could perhaps have been richer had there been more opportunity for interaction between participants. Even without convening groups of participants, I could have brought more content from previous respondents' interviews into future interviews. I tended to ask questions from my existing interview guide, which underwent only a few modifications, largely between groups, through the course of the project. The analytic benefit to consistency between individual interviews is that it enabled me to have a larger pool of data within groups, which then allowed greater comparisons between groups.

A third potential limitation concerns the extent to which I was immersed in the literature about EBM prior to conducting the interviews. Within some qualitative approaches (e.g. grounded theory), extensive knowledge of the existing literature is discouraged, in part because it positions the researcher within a particular viewpoint rather than facilitating analysis from a relatively naïve stance. This was not a grounded theory project, and within case study practice there are varying viewpoints about the extent to which one should master the existing literature. I do not think I could have conducted sufficiently sophisticated interviews without a command of the literature on EBM. Many of the arguments are too complex and intertwined with many other debates to have been able to tease them apart during hour-long interviews.

References

Bell, J. A., Hyland, S., DePellegrin, T., Upshur, R. E. G., Bernstein, M., and Martin, R. E. (2004), 'SARS and hospital priority setting: a qualitative case study and evaluation', *BMC Health Services Research*, **4** (36): 19 December <http://www.biomedcentral.com/1472-6963/4/36> accessed 6 February 2014.

Crabtree, B. F. and Miller, W. L. (1999) (eds.), *Doing qualitative research*, 2nd edn. (Thousand Oaks, CA: Sage Publications).

Creswell, J. W. (1998), *Qualitative inquiry and research design: choosing among five traditions* (Thousand Oaks, CA: Sage Publications).

Geltzer, A. (2009), 'When the standards aren't standard: evidence-based medicine in the Russian context', *Social Science in Medicine*, **68**: 526–32.

Martin, D. K., Hollenberg, D., MacRae, S., Madden, S., and Singer, P. (2003a), 'Priority setting in a hospital drug formulary: a qualitative case study and evaluation', *Health Policy*, **66**: 295–303.

Martin, D. K., Singer, P. A., and Bernstein, M. (2003b), 'Access to intensive care unit beds for neurosurgery patients: a qualitative case study', *Journal of Neurology, Neurosurgery, and Psychiatry*, **74**: 1299–303.

Sandelowski, M. (1986), 'The problem of rigor in qualitative research', *Advanced Nursing Sciences*, **8**: 27–37.

Stake, R. E. (1995), *The art of case study research* (Thousand Oaks, CA: Sage Publications).

Tiles, M. (1996), 'A science of Mars or of Venus?', in: Keller, E. F. and Longino, H. (eds.), *Feminism and science* (Oxford: Oxford University Press), 220–34.

Yin, R. K. (2003), *Case study research: design and methods*, 3rd edn. (Thousand Oaks CA: Sage Publications).

Index

A

abnormality 50, 136
absolute risk 122
ACP Journal Club 26
active ingredient 87–8, 96, 107–12
adolescent depression 140–1
affordability 28
alienists 71
Angell, M. 47, 50, 60
antidepressants
  adolescent depression 140–1
  efficacy 59–60, 110
  pragmatic trial 97
  publication bias 51
antipsychiatry movement 137–8
antipsychotics 110, 139
apotemnophilia 142–3
Ashcroft, R. E. 79, 135
auditability 192, 193
authority 19, 20, 42, 144, 160
availability 28, 123, 129
AZT 122

B

background questions 23–4, 25
behaviourist theories 76–7
Bell, J. 142
benefits 28-9
benzodiazepines 158
Berg, M. 151
best research evidence 15, 16, 17–18
  values and 118, 119–23
bias
  source of funding bias 47–51
  publication bias 47, 51–3, 140–1
  RCT design 55
  selection bias 54
  study design 27
  technical bias 55–7, 105–6
bioethicists, *see* philosophers/bioethicists
biomedical model 172
biopsychosocial model 171, 172–3
blinding 54, 95
Bluhm, R. 54
body alterations 142–3
Borgerson, K. 55
Bracken, P. 171, 173
bureaucratic tool 36–7
Burwood, S. 73
business interests 48–9, 92

C

capacity 83
Cardiac Arrhythmia Suppression Trial
  (CAST) 46, 157
case-based model 61–2
case study 188, 190
casuistic model 61–2
categorization 99–100
causal theory 74–6
Center for Drug Evaluation and Research
  (CDER) 92–3
chain sampling 190
Charles, C. 131
Charlton, B. G. 118
Chesler, P. 138
classification schemes 74–5
clinical decision analysis 22, 29, 129
clinical experience 19, 38, 80
clinical expertise 15, 28, 42, 118, 124
clinically relevant research, validity and 20
clinical observation 20
clinical questions 24
clinical trials
  commercial sponsorship 48–51,
    92, 141
  health outcomes and patient
    preferences 157
  identifying harmful drugs 31, 46, 157
  placebos 111–12
  registry 52
'clinician as perfect agent'
  decision-making 131
Cochrane Database of Systematic Reviews 25
coding 192
cognitive therapy 78
Colak, E. 61
commercially valuable interventions 48, 49
compellingness 58, 60
components of health problems 107–8
computerized decision support systems 24–5
confidence intervals 28
conflicts of interest 26, 47, 153
confounding variables 54
conscientiousness 133, 134
consequentialism 21, 128–9
consumer-survivor movement 139
controls 95
conversion disorder 77
cost issues 15, 25–6, 28, 52, 128, 130, 159
credibility 192–3

critical appraisal 22, 25, 26–9
   conflicting/insufficient data 42
   experts on 34–5, 39–40
   meaning of 'critical' 134
   responsible knowers 176
   values 120–3
   virtues 134
critical psychiatrists 139
Culpepper, L. 55

D
data
   analysis and validity 27
   becoming evidence 57–60
   collection 190
   conflicts 42
   insufficient 42
   decision board 162
decision-making 83, 84, 129, 131–2
dehumanized practice 162–3
deontological approach 128
depression
   adolescents 140–1
   criteria for 100, 142
   meaning 103–4
   subjective *vs* objective experience 105
detailing 49
diagnosis
   combinations of diagnostic criteria 99–100
   ethical controversies 135–40
   ethical framework of EBM 140–3
   in psychiatry 74–9, 85–8, 135–40
*Diagnostic and statistical manual of mental
   disorders* (DSM) 74, 76, 77, 99–100,
   138–9
diagnostic criteria
Djulbegovic, B. 135
doing mode 22
double-blind 18
Downie, R. S. 58
drug regulators 92–3
drug treatment, *see* antidepressants;
   pharmacological treatment

E
EBM developers 5
   defining EBM 32, 34
   on evidence 37
   on evidence-based psychiatry 83
   on integration 38–9
   on practice of EBM 34–5
   on values 152–3, 156, 164
educational interventions 31
effect size 27–8, 122
Elliott, C. 142
empirical observation 16
Engel, G. L. 171, 172
enlightened scepticism 15

ethical practice
   evidence-based practice and 3–4, 160–4
   psychiatric practice 170–5
ethical values
   best evidence 118, 119–23
   clinical expertise 124
   commitment of EBM 118–24
   critical appraisal 120–3
   evidence and 3, 185–6
   phases of research 3
ethics
   diagnosis and treatment 135–40
   EBM and 1–2, 91, 144
   enriched ethics of EBM 164, 165
   ethical basis of EBM 124–7
   evidence-based psychiatry 4
   psychiatric practice 170–5
   theory of ethics in evidence-based
      practice 127–31, 176-77
   trends 150–1
   values and 3–4
evidence
   best research evidence 15, 16, 17–18, 118,
      119–23
   ethical values and 3, 185–6
   evidence-based psychiatry 79–80
   expertise and 84
   experts on 37–8
   finding 24–6
   from data to 57–60
   hierarchy, *see* evidence hierarchy
   interpretation and 60
   legal notion of 58
   potential evidence 16
   'practical' 55
   primacy of 15–16
   truth and 58–9
evidence-based medicine
   applying to psychiatry 85–8
   attacks on 63
   coining of term 13
   commitment to certain ethical values 118–24
   complexity 22
   contested idea 5
   contraction 182–4
   definition 1, 13–22, 32–40
   educational interventions 31
   enriched ethics 164, 165
   epistemological assumptions 126–7
   epistemological claim 46
   ethical basis 124–7
   ethical obligation 127
   ethics and 1–2, 91
   expert definitions 32–40
   favouring pharmacological treatment 88,
      94–8
   five steps 22, 23–30, 80–2
   flexibility 164

goals 31–2, 156-8
impartiality 131
implementation 92–3
implicit values 125–6
manipulation for unethical
    purposes 117–18
medicine and 19–20
misperception 62–3
normative structure 125
online resources 2
paradigm shift 45
practice of 22–32, 34–5, 38–40
principle 1
psychiatric disorders and their
    treatments 99–107
purpose of 30–2
pursuit of health 125–6
safeguarding role 91
scope 168–70
shifting definitions 20
textbooks of 4–5, 14–15
value-free 151-2
value-laden 151-2
*Evidence-based medicine: how to practice and
    teach it* (Straus *et al*) 5, 14
    clinical expertise 118
    critical appraisal and integration 26–9,
        60–1, 63, 123
    decision analysis 129
    defining EBM 15
    educational interventions 31
    empirical observation 16
    finding evidence 24–5
    five-step process 22, 23–30
    hierarchy of research methods 18
    incorporation 26–7
    meaning of 'critical' 134
    medicine 19–20
    prognostic homogeneity 99
    question formulation 23–4
    self-evaluation 29–30, 31
    three ways of practising EBM 22–3
Evidence-Based Mental Health 25, 97–8
evidence-based practice 118–19
    ethical practice and 3–4, 160–4
    good practice and 2
    theory of ethics 127–31
evidence-based psychiatry
    critical literature 91–8
    defining 79–80
    endorsement 2–3
    ethics 4
    evidence in 79–80
    experts on 82–4
    five steps of EBM 80–2
evidence-based psychology 98
evidence hierarchy 20, 30, 41
    hierarchy of research methods 16–17

internal validity 121
psychiatry 79–80
6S hierarchy 24–5
technical bias 55–7, 105–6
values 53–7
experience of disorders 104–5
expertise 84
explanatory gap 73
external validity 55, 95–6
external values 3, 62

F
faith 36–7
Faulkner, A. 106
feasibility 28, 129
feminism 138
financial interests 60, *see also* cost issues
fittingness 192, 193
flexible evidence-based medicine 164
fluoxetine 138
follow-up studies 92
Fonagy, P. 97
foreground questions 23–4, 25
4S strategy 25
Frank, J. B. 108
Frank, J. D. 108
Fulford, K. W. M. 171, 174

G
Garland, J. 140
Geddes, J. R. 79–80
Geltzer, A. 187
Gerber, A. 118, 154
ghost writing 49
Gilbert, T. T. 55
Goldenberg, M. J. 3, 104
Goodman, K. W. 57, 168
good practice 2
GRADE system 19
Gupta, M. 134
Guyatt, G. H. 13, 135

H
happiness 128–30
harm 28, 31, 46, 139, 157
Harrison, P. J. 79–80
Haynes, B. 13, 22, 134
health, pursuit of 125–6
health outcomes
    consequentialism 128–9
    patient preferences and 156–7
Healy, D. I. 92, 140
heterogeneity 101–2
hidden values 122, 153–4
hierarchy of evidence, *see* evidence hierarchy
Holmes, J. 94
hormone replacement therapy 46
Howick, J. 55

I
impartiality 130–1
implementation 92–3
incorporation 26–7
individual clinical observation 20
individual judgement 20, 42, 61
individual patients 28–9, 60–1, 130–1
information sources, ranking 24–5
informed consent 133, 155, 193
informed decision-making 131
integration 23, 26–9, 38–9, 60–2, 63, 81
internal critique of science 191
internal validity 49, 95, 121
internal values 4
interpretation 57–60, 101–2
intuition 19, 55
involuntary hospitalization 71, 169–70,
        178, 185
involuntary treatment 139, 143, 171

J
judgement 20, 42, 55, 61
judiciousness 133

K
*Kaplan and Sadock's comprehensive textbook of
        psychiatry* (Sadock *et al*) 70, 72–3
Kesey, K. 138
Kirsch, I. 59
knowledge production 3, 47–53, 144, 165
knowledge verification 20–1
Kuhn, T. 45

L
Lauterbach, K. W. 118, 154
Lexchin, J. 51
likelihood of being helped or harm
        (LHH) 29

M
McMahon, A. D. 95
major depression, *see* depression
manual-based interventions 96
marginalization of therapies 97–8
Mathieu, S. 52
meaning, representing 103–4
meaning effect 111
mechanistic conception of body 73
medication, *see* antidepressants;
        pharmacological treatment
medicine
    EBM and 19–20
    meaning of 69
member-checking 193
mental disorder
    classification 74–5
    DSM definition 74
    notion of 70–1

mental health experts 5
    defining EBM 32–3
    on evidence 37
    on evidence-based psychiatry 84
    on political trends 150–1
    on values 153, 155, 156, 164
meta-analyses 53
mind 72–3, 77
Moerman, D. 111
Molewijk, A. C. 123
Moncrieff, J. 59, 110
multiple conditions and interventions 93

N
n-of-1 randomized trials 18, 61
non-EBM medicine 19
non-evidence-based practice 161–2
non-pharmaceutical interventions 94–8;
        see also psychotherapy
non-specific therapeutic factors 7, 88, 109-11
Norcross, J. C. 82, 98
normality 136
Nozick, R. 133
number needed to treat (NNT) 26–7

O
objective aspect of disease 104–5
objective standards 136
observational designs 55
olanzapine 93
One flew over the cuckoo's nest (Kesey) 138
opportunity cost 121
original studies 25
outcomes
    quantification 103–7
    specification 87
    see also health outcomes

P
Paris, J. 117
pathophysiologic rationale 19, 20, 61, 78–9
patient circumstances 15, 119
patient expectations 28
patient preferences 28–9, 129, 156–7
patient values 15, 28–9, 118, 119
    expert
    views 152, 154, 156
Persuasion and healing (Frank and
        Frank) 108
pharmaceutical companies
    expanding diagnostic categories 86
    source of funding bias 47, 48–51
pharmacological treatment 88, 94–8, 137, 138
philosophers/bioethicists 5
    on critical appraisal 39
    defining EBM 33, 36
    on evidence 37–8
    on evolution of EBM 40

on political trends 150–1
on values 153–4, 164
physicalists 71–4
physician values
    clinical decision-making 131–2
    expert
        views 152–3, 156
    treatment options 158
PICO format 22, 23, 24
placebos 110–12
politically important case sampling 190
political trends 150–1
Porter, R. 70
positivism 20–1
postpsychiatry 171, 173–4
post-traumatic stress disorder 142
practical evidence 55
practice of evidence-based medicine 22–32,
    34–5, 38–40
pragmatic trials 96–7
pre-appraised evidence 25, 35, 39–40, 42
precision of effect 27–8
pre-EBM medicine 19, 144
private funding 47
professional interests 50–1, 60
prognosis 85
prognostic homogeneity 99–103
propranolol 142
Prozac 138
psychiatric consumer-survivors 139
psychiatric institutions 137, 138
psychiatric practice, ethical 170–5
psychiatric symptom-rating scales 87
psychiatry
    applying EBM 85–8
    bioethics and 185–6
    case for expansion 184–5
    defining 70–9
    diagnosis and treatment 74–9, 85–8,
        99–107, 135–40
    ethical controversies 135–40
    as a legitimate medical discipline 3
    misogynistic 138
    RCTs in 92
    source of funding bias 50–1
    value-free 167–8
psychodynamic psychotherapy 56
psychological deficits 108
psychotherapy
    active ingredient 96, 109
    evaluating 94–8
    placebos 111
    practical issues 88
    shared features and functions 108–9
    theoretical pluralism 78
publication bias 47, 51–3, 140–1
public funding of research 47
pursuit of health 125–6

Q
qualitative research
    generalization 189
    on psychotherapy 97
    rigour 192–3
    technical bias 55
    Users' guides on 17
question formulation 23–4, 81

R
randomization 18, 54–5, 102–3
randomized controlled trials
    automatic privilege of 54–5
    bias 55
    flawed data from 53
    in psychiatry 92
rational practice 160, 161–2, 168, 181
'Readers' guides' series 13, 172, 173
recovery movement 139
relative risk 122
religious movement 36
replicating mode 22–3
reporting bias, *see* publication bias
research
    social context 3, 47–53
    ranking research methods 16–17, 18
resource allocation 15, 36, 118, 119, 128, 130,
        159–60, 163; *see also* cost issues
respected opinion leaders 23
responsible knowers 175–7
Reznek, L. 77
risk ratios 122
Roth, A. 97

S
Sackett, D. L. 13, 14, 159
Sadock, B. J. 70, 72–3
Sandelowski, M. 192
Schaffer, A. 103
seasonal affective disorder 75
Sehon, S. R. 63
selection bias 54
selective serotonin reuptake inhibitors 140–1
self-evaluation 29–30, 31
Shahar, E. 58
shared decision-making 131–2
shared standards 136
Showalter, E. 138
side constraints 132–3
side effects 139
6S hierarchy 24–5
size of effect 27–8, 122
social context 3, 47–53
social control 137, 138
source of funding bias 47–51
specific deficit 108, 110
Stake, R. E. 188, 189, 190
standards and standardization 136, 150, 151

Stanley, D. E. 63
STAR*D trial 97
statistical significance 122
studies 25
study design
    bias 27
    evaluation 120–1
subjective experience of disease 104–5
summaries 25
symptoms
    consistency 70
    interpretation 102
    outcome and 87, 103
    rating scales 87, 103–4
    unique/unusual 101
    weighing 124
synopses of studies 25
synopses of syntheses 25
syntheses 25
systematic reviews 18, 25
systems 24–5
systems theory 172
Szatmari, P. 117

T
technical bias 55–7, 105–6
theoretical neutrality 76–7
theoretical pluralism 78–9
therapeutic interests 48–9
Therapeutic Products Directorate of Health
    Canada 92–3
Thomas, P. 106, 171, 173
Tiles, M. 191
Timmermans, S. 151
Tonelli, M. R. 58, 61–2
treatment
    ethical controversies 135–40
    ethical framework of EBM 140–3
    physician values 158
    psychiatry 74–9, 86–8, 99–107
true knowledge 21
trust 36–7
truth 37, 58–9, 126
Turner, E. 51

U
unique symptoms 101
unsystematic clinical experience 19, 20
unusual symptoms 101
Upshur, R. E. G. 58, 61, 133, 134
user movement 139
*Users' guides to the medical literature: a manual
    for evidence-based clinical practice*
    (Guyatt *et al*) 4–5, 14

conflicting data 42
cost considerations 128, 130, 159
critical appraisal and integration 26
defining EBM 15
empirical observation 16
evidence-based practice 119
finding evidence 25–6
4S strategy 25
hierarchy of evidence 20
hierarchy of research methods 18
incorporation 26
individual patients 61
insufficient data 42
interpretation 57
medicine 19
physician values 131
primacy of evidence 15–16
publication bias 52
qualitative research 17
question formulation 24
source of funding bias 49–50
using mode 22
utilitarianism 21–2, 128, 129, 130, 134

V
validity 20, 27, 120–1
    external 55, 95–6
    internal 49, 95, 121
values 42
    diagnosis 136
    ethics and 3–4
    expert views 151–6, 164
    'hidden' 122, 153–4
    hierarchy of evidence 53–7
    implicit values of EBM 125–6
    see also ethical values; patient values;
        physician values
values-based practice 171, 174–5
verification 20–1
virtues 133–5

W
weighing options 124
weighing outcomes 103
Welsby, P. D. 93
within-category prognostic variability 100–1
Women's Health Initiative Study 46
Worrall, J. 54, 102

Y
Yin, R. K. 188, 189, 190, 192

Z
Zarkovich, E. 133